This book is due for return on or before the last date shown below.

26.10.16.

SA

AND

CHILD

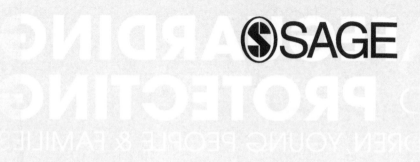

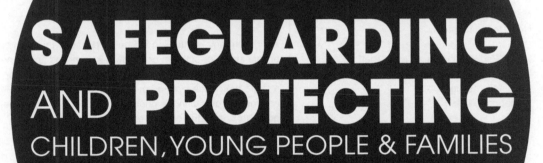

SAFEGUARDING
AND **PROTECTING**
CHILDREN, YOUNG PEOPLE & FAMILIES

A Guide for
Nurses and Midwives

Edited by

GILL WATSON & **SANDRA RODWELL**

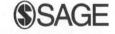

Los Angeles | London | New Delhi
Singapore | Washington DC

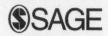

Los Angeles | London | New Delhi
Singapore | Washington DC

SAGE Publications Ltd
1 Oliver's Yard
55 City Road
London EC1Y 1SP

SAGE Publications Inc.
2455 Teller Road
Thousand Oaks, California 91320

SAGE Publications India Pvt Ltd
B 1/I 1 Mohan Cooperative Industrial Area
Mathura Road
New Delhi 110 044

SAGE Publications Asia-Pacific Pte Ltd
3 Church Street
#10-04 Samsung Hub
Singapore 049483

Editor: Becky Taylor
Associate editor: Emma Milman
Production editor: Katie Forsythe
Copyeditor: Solveig Gardner Servian
Proofreader: Thea Watson
Marketing manager: Tamara Navaratnam
Cover design: Naomi Robinson
Typeset by: C&M Digitals (P) Ltd, Chennai, India
Printed in Great Britain by Ashford Colour Press
Ltd, Gosport, Hants

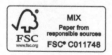
MIX
Paper from
responsible sources
FSC
www.fsc.org   FSC® C011748

Library of Congress Control Number: 2013956161

British Library Cataloguing in Publication data

A catalogue record for this book is available from
the British Library

ISBN 978-1-4462-4889-8
ISBN 978-1-4462-4890-4 (pbk)

CONTENTS

LIST OF FIGURES AND TABLES

FIGURES

TABLES

NOTES ON CONTRIBUTORS

Joan Cameron (PhD, MSc, RGN, RM) is a senior lecturer and Lead Midwife for Education at the University of Dundee. She is an experienced nurse and midwife and has extensive clinical experience of working with vulnerable women, babies and families. As an educator, she has expertise in flexible and distance learning, including developing programmes to enable nurses and midwives to implement evidence-based practice. Her research interests include caring for vulnerable infants and supporting families experiencing perinatal loss.

Jo Corlett (PhD, BA Nursing, RGN, MSc Nurse Education, RNT) has worked in a variety of clinical settings including care of the elderly, respiratory and rheumatology before completing a MSc Nurse Education at the University of Edinburgh, followed by a Registered Nurse Teacher qualification. Her first teaching position was at Abertay University in Dundee, where she remained for 10 years in various roles before moving to the University of Dundee in 2001. Since then she has been involved in the development and delivery of a variety of postgraduate programmes in various leadership roles and in 2010 was appointed as the head of the Post-Qualifying Division. Her most recent appointment is Associate Dean Head of Teaching and Learning for the School of Nursing and Midwifery. Her research interests have focused around family-centred care, safeguarding vulnerable children and families and providing parenting support. More recently research interests have focused on providing education for international students and e-learning. Jo has taught across all levels of higher education from undergraduate to PhD. Currently her main portfolio of work centres on the provision of education at post-qualifying level and in particular on meeting the academic needs of international students.

Lynn Kelly (MA (Hons), CQSW. Dip SW, MSc) qualified as a social worker in 1986 and has worked in the United Kingdom and in Australia. Lynn has been responsible for managing a wide range of multi-disciplinary teams and is interested in supervising and mentoring professionals working in the complex area of child protection. Lynn has worked mainly in the area of child protection but has also managed a large intervention service for convicted sex offenders. Lynn first joined the University of Dundee in 2004 and is currently the programme director for Child Care and Protection and the SIP Postgraduate Diploma Policing Studies. Lynn is also working to complete her doctorate and is focusing on approaches to post-qualifying education for social workers working in the child protection area.

Susan Redman (PhD, MSc, BSc, PGCert L&THE, RGN, Dip HV) is a lecturer at the School of Nursing and, Midwifery, University of Dundee. She is an experienced health visitor and has worked extensively with families to support positive parenting. Her professional areas of interest include narrative approaches to studying lives in transition, making connections between experiences of childhood and becoming a parent and media influences upon understandings of childhood. Other interests include public health within a changing global health context.

Sandra Rodwell (RNMH BSc (Health Sciences), MSc (Applied Social Research), PhD) is currently employed by NHS Tayside as a project researcher. Having originally qualified as a registered nurse in learning disabilities, she has pursued a varied career working in the voluntary and statutory sectors in the fields of direct patient care (learning disabilities and care of the elderly), development work and group advocacy (mental health) and public health (service development). Main professional areas of interest are public and client involvement in service development, public health in nursing practice and domestic abuse.

Morag Rush (MSc/PGCE, BSc, BN, PHN, RSCN, RGN) is an experienced practitioner currently working as a public health nurse/practice teacher for public health nursing students in NHS Fife. After graduating at Glasgow University she worked as a general nurse before gaining her sick children's nursing qualification at the Royal Hospital for Sick Children, Edinburgh where she worked in various roles – staff nurse, senior staff nurse and nurse specialist (wound management and plastic surgery). During that time secondment opportunities also working as a included working as a paediatric charge nurse (Perth Royal Infirmary), care co-ordination and time as a lecturer practitioner (Napier University/RHSC, Edinburgh). After training as a public health nurse (NHS Fife/Queen Margaret University) further teaching and learning experience was gained during a secondment with the University of Dundee as an associate lecturer. Currently her main interests include being a Solihull trainer and working with community partners to ensure equity of service provision and support in the community for fathers – young fathers in particular.

Gill Watson (PhD, MSc, BSc (Hons), RN, Dip HV, PGCert LandTHE). After completing her general nurse and midwifery education she worked in neonatal intensive care for a number of years in Aberdeen and in the Middle East before returning to Dundee. After completing a health visiting diploma, she worked as a generic and specialist health visitor. Her clinical experiences include working with vulnerable families: parents of very preterm infants; families infected and affected by blood-borne viruses; and people who use substances. A central part of this work involved facilitating the protection of children, and where possible, within the family environment. Much of this work involved working within a multi-professional context. Before retiring in 2013, Gill was a lecturer for 12 years in the School of Nursing and Midwifery, University of Dundee where she was responsible for leading the development of research modules for online delivery at master and degree levels. She also contributed to the development of programmes for both undergraduate and postgraduate students. Since her retirement, Gill has developed a motivational business incorporating hypnosis as an approach to supporting behavioural change.

FOREWORD

I am delighted to be writing a foreword to this most timely publication.

The early years are critical in shaping health and wellbeing throughout life (DH 2013: 2). Providing safe, effective and evidence-based care and ensuring positive outcomes for infants, children, young people and families are essential. In line with all UK policy relating to early years, the roles of nurses, health visitors, midwives and school nurses are highlighted as paramount in ensuring proactive, early identification, assessment and intervention for all women and families (Cowley et al. 2013, DH 2011). In partnership with many other groups and agencies these professionals also contribute to addressing the wider public health agenda by: undertaking work with individuals, groups or communities; providing specialist input to vulnerable populations such as looked after and excluded children and to families where issues such as domestic abuse, mental health or substance misuse exist.

Emerging evidence shows that early intervention and support is key to helping children reach their full potential. Achieving the best possible start requires intervention from highly trained and skilled nurses and professionals.

This text concentrates on the early years of life. It provides guidance on attachment, risk, safeguarding, vulnerability, parenting, domestic abuse and to engaging and working with children, young people and families. As an experienced nurse, health visitor, manager and consultant I have watched support provided to patients and families change and develop over the years as it has adapted to new knowledge, changes in public expectations and changes in the way services are delivered. The need for nurses and professionals to understand attachment, the theory and evidence on which to base decisions, the context and challenges in providing care and how early infant and child development can be both promoted and damaged is essential.

The selection of subject areas in this book is commendable. The use of questions, case studies and reflective activity make strong illustrations and arguments about the nature of policy, theory and practice and their collective importance. The text is a welcome contribution to understanding the importance of providing family-centred care and provides an intelligent platform to inform students and future leaders, particularly those drawn from clinical professions and practice. The current climate in healthcare realises the importance of early years and therefore this book could not be more timely. For those nurses, midwives, health visitors and allied health professionals wishing to increase their knowledge or work with infants, children or families this text will provide stimulation, debate and a credible source of reference.

Dr Julia Egan
Consultant in Public Health Nursing, NHS Tayside.

REFERENCES

Cowley.S., Whittaker.K., Grigulis.A., Malone.M., Donetto.S., Wood.H., Morrow.E., Maben.J. (2013) *Why Health Visiting? A Review of the Literature about Key Health Visitor Interventions, Processes and Outcomes for Children and Families* (Department of Health Policy Research programme, ref. 016 0058). London: Kings College.

Department of Health (2011) *Health Visitor Implementation Plan 2011–15: A Call to Action*. February. London: Department of Health.

Department of Health (2013) *The National Health Visitor Plan: Progress to Date and Implementation 2013 Onwards*. London: Department of Health.

INTRODUCTION

GILL WATSON AND SANDRA RODWELL

The contribution of healthcare professionals towards protecting children and young people has expanded significantly over the last 10 years. This change has not occurred in isolation but within the context of evolving social and healthcare policies to address children's rights within the United Kingdom. The changing face of child protection in healthcare within the United Kingdom has highlighted the need to develop this book as an introduction to safeguarding children and young people.

Nursing and midwifery practitioners form a large percentage of the healthcare workforce (Sharp 2012). Through their respective professional caring roles nurses and midwives have access to a large number of patients, or clients, including infants, children, young people and adults across a range of specialties and spanning all healthcare environments. Regulatory bodies, such as the Nursing and Midwifery Council (NMC) and in the case of dental nurses the General Dental Council (GDC), state clearly the need for accountability and responsibility in relation to advocacy, confidentiality and disclosure of risk of individuals who are being maltreated. Legislation, policy and the professional regulation leave nursing and midwifery practitioners in no doubt as to their responsibilities towards individual infants/children/young people who are judged to be potentially or at actual risk of harm or causing harm to others.

The context in which healthcare is organised and delivered in both primary, secondary or private healthcare within the United Kingdom means that there are times or situations when children and their families may be cared for by nursing practitioners other than those trained specifically to care for children. Safeguarding children therefore becomes every practitioners' business and not just those working directly with children. This is important for those working within adult nursing services, including mental health and drug and alcohol services. As Cuthbert and Stanley remind us:

> Adult-focused services addressing problems such as domestic abuse, drug and alcohol abuse and mental illness often fail to recognise that their clients are parents as well. (2012: 243)

Therefore all practitioners are now required to be aware, not only of the client or patient they have direct contact with but also of others such as an unborn infant,

infant, child or young person who may be at risk of harm. Practitioners also need to be aware of their role in child protection and what this means in practical terms in their sphere of practice.

For healthcare managers, health boards and authorities across the United Kingdom, preparing nurses and midwives to meet safeguarding policies through their daily practice is a significant activity to undertake. Policies across all four nations have set out standards of practice relating to all universal services and not just social care alone. The message from policy is clear and explicit. Healthcare practitioners, along with other professionals, need to apply a set of specific safeguarding standards in their daily practice. However, there is evidence to suggest that the practices of nurses and midwives have been slow to respond to the safeguarding needs of children and young people.

ABOUT THIS BOOK

This book has been developed for undergraduate and postgraduate nurses and midwives. It is not a comprehensive guide but offers an introduction to safeguarding and the protection of children and young people and their families for nurses and midwives. The contents may also serve as a resource for those already working in practice. Other professional disciplines may want to use this text as a source of reference in relation to their own practice.

AIMS OF THIS BOOK

The presentation and content of this introductory text is guided by three broad aims. The first is to introduce the main theories used to inform child safeguarding and protection practices. Knowledge and understanding of specific theories are required by individual nurses and midwives, as well as other multi-professional practitioners. The second aim is to support on-going development of the necessary knowledge and skills needed to support the application of interventions which best safeguard and protect children and their families. Interventions in this context refer to all the tasks most likely to be used in order to identify, prevent and reduce significant harm in the lives of children and young people. The final aim is to raise awareness about the level of support required by practitioners in order that they are effective in their child safeguarding role.

THE CONTENT

We acknowledge at this point that all children and young people require safeguarding as well as protection from harm. However, much of the underlying theory addresses early years development of children. This is to highlight the significance of development within the first three years of a young child's life and the long-term impact this early stage may have on later development.

A further point to raise is that the content is prepared to address the need to safeguard and protect not only children and young people, but also the families in which they develop. For the majority of children, the family environment is where they will spend a lot of time. While it is acknowledged that many family environments may be considered or assessed as less than optional, it is unlikely in most cases that the child or children would be removed unless considered absolutely necessary. Practitioners, more than ever before, are required to work with families in order to improve the home environment, supporting child welfare and reducing the risk of significant harm. This book therefore addresses safeguarding children and young people, as well as the family, through prevention and reducing harm.

Following this introduction, this book is presented in three parts. The first part, entitled *Policies and theories*, consists of four chapters, each of which addresses a theoretical approach aligned to contemporary child care policies and which inform the practices of all universal services, including nursing and midwifery services. The reason for including specific theories relates to the evidence which highlights that nurses have reported feeling unprepared to fulfil their roles and responsibilities towards safeguarding activities as well as lacking in confidence.

Chapter 1, *Policy to practice*, provides a brief historical account of social policy and how it is developed. The impact of the media in child protection matters and the influence of the United Nations Convention on the Rights of the Child (UNCRC) (1989) are discussed. A further point addressed in this chapter is a discussion on the approach adopted to deliver contemporary child care policies. It is here that the public health approach is highlighted before exploring the application of competency frameworks to ensure that nurses and midwives are sufficiently prepared with the knowledge and skills to fulfil contemporary child care policies.

Chapter 2, *Key themes in safeguarding and protecting children and young people*, introduces the key concepts of child abuse and neglect. A summary of the incidence and prevalence of child abuse and neglect in the lives of children living in the four nations is provided. A number of key points around the role of nurses and midwives are introduced. This chapter lays the foundation for the wide-ranging discussions running through this book.

Chapter 3, *Attachment*, explores theories which inform understanding of how infants develop attachments to their parents and the impact this relationship has on the first three years of the developing young child. Knowledge and understanding of attachments, how they form and the influence of sensitive parenting on the quality of the attachment are needed when assessing conditions which may or may not contribute to risk.

The final chapter in part one is Chapter 4, *Risk assessment*, which explores the main aspects of risk assessment and management. The main processes of risk management are discussed, as are the activities and structures which can impact on the overall quality of assessing risk and decision making. Central to this chapter is the assessment framework as well as the tools to support assessment and decision making.

Part two, entitled *Relationships, communication and practice*, contains a further four chapters exploring aspects of communication and how this can influence the formation of relationships between children, their families and practitioners. Chapter 5, *Vulnerability in pregnancy and childbirth*, examines the impact of social vulnerability and the risks imposed through social exclusion. While this chapter focuses on pregnancy and midwifery practice, it has much to offer other practitioners working in healthcare.

Chapter 6, *Supporting the development of positive parenting*, explores the implications of contemporary social policy on parenting, raising questions around the need to support parents to fulfil their roles and responsibilities through the provision of sensitive care. Contemporary literature is discussed and case studies from the Family Nurse Partnership project, the Solihull Parenting Programme and Triple P are presented. Theoretically, the discussion is underpinned with reference to 'recognition and reciprocity' as fundamental to sensitive parenting and meeting the public health agenda for safeguarding children and supporting parents. This chapter provides a pragmatic approach as to how well parents can be supported in practice.

In Chapter 7 the philosophy and concept of *Family-centred care* is explored from a historical perspective as well as through a review of present day literature. The United Nations Convention on the Rights of the Child identifies explicitly the importance of parents in the lives of children. The importance of parenting becomes more significant when for the first time parenting responsibilities and rights are identified in the Children Act (1989 and 2004) and the Children (Scotland) Act (1995). While family-centred care has been around for some time within health and social care, the degree to which it has been applied in practice has been variable. This chapter explores the factors that influence the quality of therapeutic partnerships between parents and nursing staff. Of particular significance is the influence of professional power and how it can be applied and used more positively in practice through communication and meaningful interaction.

Chapter 8 explores the important role of practitioners *Engaging with children, young people and their families*. Practitioners working with children, young people and their families have a responsibility to ensure that all situations are explained in full to ensure understanding and reduce uncertainty. However, many children continue to be ignored. It is crucial that children and young people have the opportunity to tell of their experience and participate in any decision making regarding their situation and future management, and made to feel part of the team. The developmental stage of each child needs to be considered when preparing to interact and communicate. Frameworks to aid the communication process and to ensure that the gathering of experiences are recorded and reported to the wider inter-disciplinary team are introduced and discussed.

The third and final part addresses *Factors impacting on practice*, and comprises two chapters, each addressing issues that impact on nursing and midwifery practice. Chapter 9, *Responding to domestic abuse in the lives of children*, addresses domestic abuse but not through conventional means. The findings from research exploring the views and experiences of nurses and midwives working in a community setting and their response to children living with domestic abuse form the basis of this chapter, which is presented in three parts. This chapter has much to offer not only practitioners but also their managers and educators through raising many of the issues that are often discussed in private but without acknowledgement from more formal support systems.

Chapter 10, *Getting it right: supporting professional responses to child safeguarding and protection*, discusses the emerging themes from the preceding chapters which were considered relevant in the preparation of nursing and midwifery practitioners to safeguard and protect children, young people and their families. Practice development, conceptualised using an ecological framework, is presented as a means of addressing the present day limitations in nursing and midwifery practice.

APPLYING A REFLECTIVE APPROACH

The movement towards graduate nursing and midwifery education requires practitioners to have and to apply and use analysis and critical thinking in their practice. Reflection and reflective activities, such as critical reflection and synthesis of evidence (Duke and Appleton 2008), are considered central to problem solving and decision making, contributing to learning in clinical practice and the facilitation of professional development (Gustafsson 2004). To support learning in this way, reflective activities along with other learning tasks, such as case histories, are included in many of the chapters. Regardless of the learning activities, active reflection is part of the developmental process.

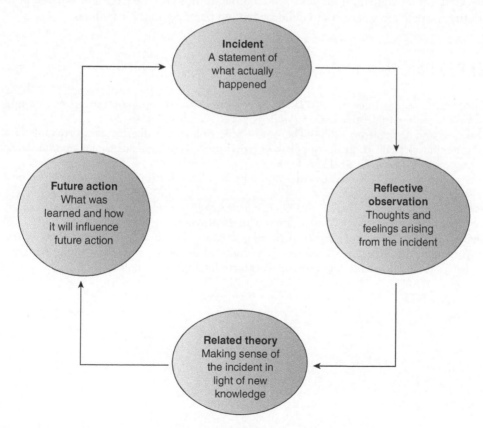

Figure 0.1   Reflection cycle (Marks-Maran and Rose 1997)

While many students and other readers may have a preference for a specific reflective model to guide the reflective process, others may not. To aid the latter we have included an example of Marks-Maran and Rose's (1997) Reflection Cycle in Figure 0.1, accompanied by a brief explanation of the four common interactive processes.

In reference to the reflective activities, 'the incident' commonly refers to your experiences gained in clinical practice. Once identified, consider your 'reflective observations' of the incident, taking note of the resulting thoughts and feelings which you experienced in relation to the incident you are being asked to consider. Next, consider what you need to learn. This is identifying 'related theory'. Some of this detail may well be located within the book; however, you may find it useful to search out other resources to inform your thinking. Finally, consider what you have learnt following the reflective activity and how will this inform any 'future action'. This point is important because you may then need to return to work through the reflection cycle once again after reviewing any changes in your practice.

All contributors to this book have experience of practice in health and/or social care as well as having contributed in the academic development of others. Such experiences are vital if their contributions are to be credible to those on the front line with responsibility for delivering services to children, young people and their families.

REFERENCES

Cuthbert, C. and Stanley, K. (2012) All babies count: a new approach to prevention and protection for vulnerable babies. *Public Policy Research* 184: 243–247.

Duke, S. and J. Appleton (2008) The use of reflection in a palliative care programme: a quantitative study of the development of reflective skills over an academic year. *Journal of Advanced Nursing* 32(6): 1557–1568.

Gustafsson, C. (2004) Reflection, the way to professional development? *Journal of Clinical Nursing* 13(3): 271–280.

Marks-Maran, D. and Rose, P. (1997) *Reconstructing Nursing: Beyond Art and Science*. London: Bailliere Tindall in association with the Royal College of Nursing.

Sharp, B. (2012) The role of nurses in delivering integrated healthcare: workforce implications. Reshaping the Nursing Workforce: preparing professionals for new working patterns. King's Fund Presentation, Centre for Workforce Intelligence, London.

PART 1

POLICIES AND THEORIES

1

POLICY TO PRACTICE

LYNN KELLY, GILL WATSON AND SANDRA RODWELL

CHAPTER SUMMARY

Policy is intrinsically related to practice. Policies guide the direction and capacity of practice by setting out clearly expected standards of practice to meet policy outcomes. Health and social care policies are wide ranging and generally informed and developed from an eclectic evidence base, for example national and localised statistics, service user experiences, policy reviews and academic research.

Social welfare policies, encompassing health and social care, inform what are referred to as the universal services, commonly including health, social, educational services and law enforcement. The nature of policies addressing childhood and the family is subject to the changing philosophical, political and moral codes of the day, thus evolving over time to what society perceives acceptable at a specific point in history. The construction of childhood, adolescence and family life in society is frequently challenged within private, social and political arenas and remains the most heavily contested area of social welfare policy in the United Kingdom today.

Over the last 20-year period there has been increased media reporting of high-profile child deaths resulting from abuse and neglect. In many of those cases parental and organisational factors have been uncovered as contributing to child deaths. Organisational failings such as poor leadership and management and limited resources as well poor frontline practices have been identified as compounding vulnerable familial environments with poor outcomes for children.

Nonetheless, as child social welfare policies have evolved so too have the practices of frontline practitioners in both social and health care to reflect the changing status of children in society. Central to policy changes is the status of children as active citizens, actively contributing to decisions about their lives. It is important to consider the relationship between social welfare policy and healthcare practice and how this has influenced individual and inter-professional working in the provision of services for children.

This chapter will address the influences on the development of social welfare policy relating to child welfare such as the rights-based agenda, legislative and policy environment and evidence-based interventions. This chapter concludes by reflecting on emerging themes and challenges for the future.

AIMS OF THIS CHAPTER

Following a brief outline of the historical context in which social welfare policy has evolved, this chapter has two aims. The first aim is to consider the most significant influences on policy and practice, including international conventions and legislation. The second aim is to examine the public health approach used to deliver contemporary child social welfare policy and the preparation of practitioners and health and social care organisations to contribute to meeting policy outcomes relating to child welfare.

Learning outcomes

After reading this chapter and following a period of reflection the reader will be able to:

- Analyse critically the political and social context in which child social welfare and protection professionals operate in the United Kingdom.
- Reflect critically on the quality and adequacy of the response of individual practitioners, organisations and society to safeguarding and protecting children.
- Consider critically the use of the public health approach to delivering contemporary child social welfare policy.
- Analyse critically the preparation of all practitioners to fulfil their roles and responsibility to meet contemporary child social welfare policy.

Key words

child protection; child safeguarding; child welfare; interventions; legislation; policy; political ideology; public health

WHAT IS MEANT BY SOCIAL WELFARE POLICY?

Social welfare policy is the means by which national and local governments set out objectives to meet the welfare, sometimes referred to as social, needs of the population. Within the United Kingdom social policies address education, health, housing, social security and occasionally law and order (Marshall 1998). Much of social policy is organised around the social unit of the family who, until the last century, bore much of the responsibility for the provision of child welfare and protection. However, over the last 100 years, national and local governments have accepted greater responsibilities for child welfare.

The link between child welfare and child protection has not always been transparent. Indeed, until the start of the 21st century child protection was most often aligned to the justice system while child welfare was considered as something quite separate. Child protection was identified as a narrow field, disconnected from other aspects of childhood and the ecology of family life. More recently child protection was recognised as being nested within, and intrinsic to, the welfare of the child (Vincent 2010). Incorporating the welfare and protection of children as one concept by policy makers has widened understanding of the needs of children and increased the responsibilities of a wider welfare workforce to meet children's needs. It was at this time when safeguarding came to be viewed as the all-inclusive umbrella term given to the totality of child welfare and protection. It is important, however, to consider some of the principle historical milestones which have contributed to social welfare policy today.

HISTORICAL SOCIAL WELFARE POLICY MILESTONES IMPACTING ON CHILD WELFARE AND PROTECTION

The English Poor Law was established in 1601 but continued right through in one form or another until 1948. The Poor Law represented what is known as a 'residual model' of welfare. That is, welfare provision for those with nowhere else to turn and no longer able to provide for themselves or their families. The Poor Law was intended to be punitive and to act as a deterrent. Later, an alternative perspective on welfare was considered that took the view that need and dependency were normal conditions in society. This model of welfare is referred to as the 'institutional model' (Spicker 2008). It is on the values of this institutional model of welfare that our present welfare state is based. The Report of the Inter-Departmental Committee on Social Insurance and Allied Services (1942), known more commonly as the Beveridge Report, was an influential document in the founding of the welfare state in the United Kingdom (Beveridge 1942). This report identified five 'giant evils' in society – squalor, ignorance, want, idleness and disease – and went on to propose widespread reform to the system of social welfare to address these evils. This report is commonly acknowledged to be the foundation of the welfare state and subsequently the National Health Service as we understand it today. The focus of this report was to ensure that citizens were healthy enough to contribute to the economic growth of the United Kingdom. It is interesting to note that children were not viewed with any significance at this time.

Reflective activity

Reflecting upon the five 'great evils' identified by the Beveridge Report (1942), what are the 'great evils' facing us today? Are there any differences?

Following on from Beveridge (1942), two international conventions had a significant influence on contemporary child welfare policies: the United Nations Convention on the Rights of the Child (UNCRC) (1989) and the European Convention on Human Rights (ECHR) (1950). Together, these conventions have informed what is referred to as the rights-based agenda.

Rights-based agenda

In 1991 the government of the United Kingdom ratified and signed up to the UNCRC (1989). In the United Nations Convention on the Rights of the Child (1989) Article 19 sets out the duty of governments to protect children from all forms of violence and abuse by taking the required measures, be they legal, educational, social or administrative. This obligation applies to all children whether they are living with their parents, are looked after or are being cared for by some other arrangement. At the same time the UNCRC (1989) also promotes the importance of the family as the best form of protection for children. Providing appropriate support to families is proffered as a means of ensuring that the rights of children are respected (Henricson and Bainham 2005). While not denying the individual rights of the child, the underlying message to governments set out in the UNCRC (1989) is that policies should reflect the interdependency of families and consider the rights of children within this context and not in isolation (Henricson and Bainham 2005). There is, however, a danger that by focusing on the child within the family situation, responding to the broader issues that are impacting on the family situation may take precedence. In these situations the individual needs of the child may then be lost among the needs of the adults and the family as a whole (Henricson and Bainham 2005).

Within the United Kingdom, the government is also bound by the European Convention on Human Rights (ECHR 1950). The principles set out in ECHR (1950) are set out in the Human Rights Act (1998) in the United Kingdom (HM Government 1998). While the ECHR (1950) does not make specific reference to children, both adults and children have rights within this convention (Henricson and Bainham 2005). Article 3 states that 'no one shall be subject to torture or to inhuman or degrading treatment or punishment' (ECHR 1950), while Article 8 (which is in two parts) states that 'everyone has the right to respect for his private and family life, his home and his correspondence' (ECHR 1950). The second part cautions against undue interference by the authorities unless for reasons stated in Article 8(2), which relate to national interest as well as situations when other individuals' freedoms and rights are compromised (ECHR 1950). The ECHR (1950) requires governments and service providers to perform a balancing act in order that they do not breach their obligations, particularly with respect to Articles 3, 8(1) and 8(2). Accusations of failure to protect, in line with Article 3, may be levelled at those who know that a child is in need of protection but are found to have not done enough to protect that child. Conversely, if efforts to protect a child are too zealous then an infringement of the human rights of parents may be the charge under Article 8(2); the rights of parents cannot be ignored (Henricson and Bainham 2005).

The rights-based agenda directed through two significant international conventions required governments, organisations and individual practitioners to undertake their duties with respect for the rights of families and individuals within families, be they parents, children or other family members, and not to interfere unduly (Roberts 2001, Lowden 2002, Henricson and Bainham 2005). It is important to note that the notion of what constitutes a family continues to be debated within legal, political and academic settings both within the European Union and the United Kingdom. The government however continues to emphasise the importance of the family with two parents being considered as the key source of welfare and care for children (Roberts 2001). This approach is in accordance with the UNCRC (1989), which also promotes support for the family as the main means of ensuring that the rights of children are upheld (Henricson and Bainham 2005).

Within the United Kingdom many organisations and policy documents focused on children draw on the series of wide reaching statements contained within the UNCRC (1989) and the ECHR (1950) as a means of giving authority to what they do (Foley et al. 2001). While reflecting concern for the welfare of children and issues pertaining to child protection, the principles laid out in the UNCRC (1989) are also aimed at giving children the status of citizenship. This move promotes and supports the view that children who are able to form and give an opinion should have the opportunity to express their views with respect to decisions which affect them, as stated in Article 12 of the UNCRC (1989). The United Kingdom sets out to meet its international obligations through the Human Rights Act 1998 and a number of legislative measures reflecting the principle of placing the welfare and best-interests of children and young people at the centre of policy and practice (Foley et al. 2001; Scottish Executive 2001; Department for Education and Skills 2004).

POLITICAL DEVELOPMENTS IN THE UNITED KINGDOM AND THE SOCIAL WELFARE AGENDA SINCE BEVERIDGE

The Thatcher government of 1979–90 marked the period where United Kingdom turned away from the Beveridge vision of welfare back to a more 'residual', also referred to as neo-liberal, model particularly in relation to social welfare, education, health and community care. At the core of this thinking was the belief that citizens should be responsible for their own welfare and that the State should only intervene as a last resort. In all but exceptional circumstances, individuals should be free to choose the services they require from a range of providers. Health and social care now operated within the concept of a 'free market'. Large-scale privatisation of welfare provision in the United Kingdom took place over this period with a strong emphasis on individualism and responsibility towards immediate family and the wider community, theoretically providing the individual with greater choice.

Reflective activity

Reflecting on the principles underpinning social welfare policy development during the Thatcher administration, what provision was made for supporting child welfare?

Interestingly, it was during Conservative rule that legislation in the form of the Children Act (1989) in England, also influencing Wales and Northern Ireland, and the Children (Scotland) Act (1995) were passed, underpinned by the rights-based agenda. Yet there was little change in policy direction until Labour's 'third way' set the new policy direction towards what we have today.

New Labour: the third way

The United Kingdom electorate rejected neo-liberal ideals and in 1997 the Blair government was elected on a wave of popularity. Under the leadership of Tony Blair the Labour Party reinvented itself as 'New Labour' and claimed to be seeking a new way of governing called the 'third way', viewed as the middle ground between the extremes of neo-liberalism and the post-war welfare state. This new government moved away from developing policies influenced by economics alone towards policies shaped by dimensions of social and economic integration. Equally important at this time were the values placed on equality and opportunities. Hence we witnessed the drive towards social inclusion policies which embrace social investment, participation and reducing inequalities with the potential of improving the quality of life for children and their families.

The move towards addressing inequalities

Wide-ranging policy changes across many areas impacting on health and social care were initiated by New Labour. The independent inquiry into inequalities in health resulted in the Acheson Report (1998). Reducing inequalities was central in all other policy areas in order that inequalities in health could be reduced. While the Acheson Report (1998) has received some criticism for not sufficiently prioritising changes, Sir Donald Acheson did contribute to the on-going re-establishment of the public health movement in contemporary politics.

A further initiative set up by New Labour was the development of the Social Exclusion Unit (SEU) in 1998 to address what were termed 'deprived neighbourhoods' made up of housing estates with significant problems of unemployment, drug use, crime, poor housing and breakdown in community cohesion. The report *Bringing Britain Together* (Social Exclusion Unit 1998) identified that previous social and economic policies had contributed to the breakdown in these neighbourhoods. This and further analysis resulted in the *National Strategy Action Plan* (Social Exclusion Unit 2001) to refocus social and economic resources to improve housing, reduce crime, reduce unemployment and generally re-establish community cohesion through empowerment. Social policies at this time viewed children as a valuable asset for future human investment.

Child welfare

The children's rights framework (UNCRC 1989) and the Human Rights Act (1998) started to emerge as influencing child welfare policies. During the Labour government new policy direction contributed towards the movement from narrow child protection policies to much wider, all-inclusive child welfare and safeguarding policies (Vincent 2010). The changes in healthcare policy reflected the wider social and economic developments. A significant report regarding healthcare followed the Bristol Inquiry into the deaths of children following heart surgery in Bristol Royal Infirmary reinforced and supported the need for changes to health services for children (Kennedy 2001). Following the changes in healthcare for children and young people came the creation of a parliamentary minister (Member of Parliament) with responsibility for children and young people while a Children's Commissioner Office was established across the four nations. Starting in the early years of the 21st century, contemporary child welfare policies adopted a much wider approach to safeguarding children rather than the narrower focus of child protection.

Present-day political picture

Britain's welfare system today represents an interesting mix of principles and influences as the General Election of 2010 did not return a majority government. The Conservatives and Liberal Democrats entered into a formal coalition agreement, the first of its kind for 60 years. Despite declared differences between the two parties, the unifying issue of the coalition has been the need to tackle the fallout from the worldwide economic crisis of 2007–2010.

There is still a relatively strong foundation of welfare state principles. However, in this present climate of challenging fiscal demands, the level of support given to address the welfare needs of children and their families appears to be reducing. Successive governments have failed to reduce child poverty; relative poverty continues to be problematic for one in four children. Child poverty therefore remains problematic in the United Kingdom and is an area which needs to be addressed by concurrent effective policies.

Reflective activity

What has the coalition administration done to address child welfare since coming into power?

The development of effective policies is directed by a legislative framework.

LEGISLATIVE FRAMEWORK OF CHILD WELFARE

The key legislation informing child protection policy and practice in the United Kingdom today is presented in Figures 1.1 and 1.2. There is not one single piece of legislation which addresses child protection in entirety within the United Kingdom. However, there are a number of legislative acts which have been amended, updated and revoked (NSPCC 2011). Devolution has required all four nations within the United Kingdom to develop separate legislation for the protection of children based on the same principles as set out in the United Nations Convention on the Rights of the Child (1989) and the European Convention of Human Rights (1950). Although they are not legislative acts, conventions are powerful bodies in their own right. The Human Rights Act (1998) also contributed to the principled framework underpinning legislation within and across the United Kingdom.

The Children Act 1989

The Children (Scotland) Act 1995

The Children (Northern Ireland) Order 1995

The Human Rights Act 1998

The Children's Commissioner Acts in England, Wales, Scotland and Northern Ireland in 2001 and 2003

The Children Act (2004)

The Safeguarding Vulnerable Groups Act 2006

The Protection of Vulnerable Groups (Scotland) Act 2007

Figure 1.1   Legislation informing the protection of children

Legislation that protects children and young people from adults who pose a risk to them includes:

The Children and Young Persons Act 1933

The Sex Offenders Act 1997

Figure 1.2 Legislation informing child protection from adults who pose a risk

National reports, reviews and inquiries have a significant impact on the development and implementation of policy into practice, providing a governance function.

National reports, reviews and inquiries into child welfare policy

Two significant reports from within the United Kingdom contributed to social welfare policy development. The first was the audit and review of child protection services within Scotland in 2002. The second report was the inquiry into the death of Victoria Climbié chaired by Lord Laming and published in January 2003. Both had a significant impact on national child protection policy and practice.

The audit and review of child protection services in Scotland resulted in the report *It's Everyone's Job to Make Sure I'm Alright* (Scottish Executive 2002). While areas of good practice were identified, the review panel also illuminated areas of 'significant weaknesses'. The findings led to far-reaching changes in the delivery of children's services in all aspects of health, education and social care in Scotland (*Getting it Right for Every Child*, Scottish Executive 2005) (Vincent 2010). The Laming Inquiry informed the development of wide-reaching child safeguarding policies in England and Wales (*Every Child Matters*, Department for Education and Skills 2003) and more recently in England (*Working Together to Safeguard Children*, Department for Education 2013); Northern Ireland (*Our Children and Young People – Our Shared Responsibility: The Reform Implementation Process in Child Protection Services in Northern Ireland*, Social Services Inspectorate 2006) (Social Services Inspectorate 2006); and in Wales following devolution (*Children and Young People: Rights to Action*, Welsh Assembly Government 2004).

While conventions, political ideology, legislation and a robust evidence base shape policy and practice, the media also reflects and influences societal attitudes.

Influence of the media

The general public also influenced contemporary child social welfare policy development through multi-media outlets which undoubtedly had a significant role in allowing individuals to express concerns and thoughts which ultimately contributed to forming and influencing the attitudes and behaviour of others. Cunningham and Cunningham (2012) reported 800 'substantive' articles in the United Kingdom press about child abuse from July 2010 to July 2011 and the Baby Peter case resulted in over 2,500 articles.

Many of the media reports reviewed appeared to focus mainly on high-profile cases which, in many instances, involved the death of a child. However, these media reports can at times fail to provide a balanced view and invite an emotional reaction, leading to much criticism of professionals responsible for delivering child welfare services. The public are not always aware of all the circumstances which may have a detrimental impact on individual practitioners and the discipline they belong to, for example nurses, doctors, social workers, midwives.

Reflective activity

When considering the detail of media reports into child maltreatment, can you identify what factors are reported more frequently and what factors are often missing?

While criticism of practitioners is warranted in some cases, as reported by Lord Laming following the inquiry into the death of Victoria Climbié (Laming 2003) and the audit and review into child protection (Scottish Executive 2002) in Scotland, there are often other contributing factors which are not reported, such as the unacceptable levels of socioeconomic disadvantage frequently found contributing in some capacity to poor levels of child welfare, or the cut-back in the number of practitioners supporting families.

Reflective activity

How can media reports of child maltreatment provide a more balanced picture of events?

NEW POLICY: A PUBLIC HEALTH APPROACH

Refocusing on child welfare policy has moved away from children 'at risk' of maltreatment towards a much wider focus, therefore the development of contemporary child care policies and practices have changed. Identifying children and families in need of support became the mantel in contemporary policy design, thereby supporting prevention as well as reducing the possibility of abuse and neglect from taking place. This crucial change in child welfare policy needed to be all-encompassing and child-centred while at the same time reaching out to every child and family; not just those deemed to be at risk of harm. Policies therefore needed to direct practice and practitioners to adopt a change in approach.

The discipline of Public Health has addressed a number of health and social problems impacting on populations such as housing, education, employment and law enforcement. In his Foreword introducing *Public Health for the 21st Century*,

Professor Mike Kelly stated that 'Public health has always been political and has always been multi disciplinary' (2003).

A significant advantage of using a public health approach rests with the use of a conceptual framework which provides a systematic means of assessing populations and developing actions and policies to meet child safeguarding policy outcomes. The approach recognises that child maltreatment is indeed preventable through addressing the risks that contribute to child abuse and neglect, through the introduction of early interventions and multi-professional involvement requiring the engagement of services beyond healthcare (Miller 2003; Scally 2003).

The breadth of the approach transcends other policy areas known to impact on health (Frieden 2010). A public health approach has the ability to impact on the wider social welfare policy agenda influencing the determinants which create healthier lives. Two distinct levels of interventions are noted in the social welfare policy guidance across the United Kingdom: universal and targeted interventions

Universal or targeted interventions

One of the biggest changes in practice, especially for health and educational services, is the introduction of universal and targeted interventions. While this approach was instigated some years before, healthcare services appeared reluctant to become fully involved.

Universal services are those services which are accessible to all children and families. This approach provides a baseline service to all at specific and identified times. In the main, universal provision is the domain of healthcare and educational practitioners. Healthcare is the front-line universal intervention provider for preschool children with the family health visitor recognised as the child/children's named nurse. For children attending school, universal interventions are provided via educational services. For children with changing needs, other interventions can be introduced by involving other agencies (Vincent and Daniel 2010). One strength of universal services provision is that children requiring greater interventions are not passed from one service to another with a possibility of being 'lost' in the process. A further strength is the involvement of healthcare and educational services as the main providers of universal interventions, therefore leaving social workers to target children with the greatest need (Vincent and Daniel 2010).

There are concerns, however, regarding the ability of services to deliver. The evidence supporting the effectiveness of universal provision, in general and also in children's' services, is insufficient (Baker 2011) and more research is required to identify the efficacy of such an approach. Compounding the lack of evidence relating to the efficacy of universal services is the level and quality of preparation given to those providing such services. Munro (2011) highlights that those providing children's services do not as yet have the relevant competencies to commit fully to their safeguarding roles. While Munro made these comments in relation to universal services, there is evidence which suggests that nurses are not confident or prepared to participate in the protection of children. This situation is a concern. In his report following the Victoria Climbié Inquiry, Lord Laming stated:

There is a huge task to be undertaken to ensure that in each of the services, staff are trained adequately to carry out their duties in the care and protection of children and support to families. A balance between theoretical teaching and practical training should be guaranteed on all training courses. All staff appointed to any of the services where they will be working with children and families must have adequate training for the positions they will fill. However, along with this general requirement of competence to do the job, it is vital that all staff have the benefit of a period of induction that covers, specifically, their roles in protecting children and supporting families. (2003: 11)

Early interventions are considered to be the benchmark of good practice. The use of the term 'early interventions' is perhaps ambiguous; however, a helpful definition of early intervention is offered by the Centre for Excellence and Outcomes in Children and Young People's Services (C4EO):

Intervening early and as soon as possible to tackle problems emerging for children, young people and their families or with a population most at risk of developing problems. Early interventions may occur at any point in a child or young person's life. (2011: 4)

The *Early Intervention: The Next Step* report (Allen 2011) highlights the need for early interventions at different stages in the child's life to develop what he terms their 'foundation years'. However, early interventions are also those interventions used to prevent reoccurrence of conditions leading to poor welfare and development, or worse still maltreatment. Early interventions contribute to limiting long-term impairment.

According to Munro (2011) it is this level of early intervention which is central to delivering contemporary child safeguarding policy. The focus of early interventions is therefore to identify and prevent risk factors recognised as contributing to child maltreatment from impacting negatively on the developing child. However, there is an argument that there is also a need for early interventions to reduce and prevent on-going distress if maltreatment has already occurred, to prevent further on-going abuse, recurrence and long-term impairment. The main focus of early interventions is therefore to reduce risk of harm or indeed reduce the impact of further harm occurring once maltreatment has taken place.

Targeted interventions are more commonly required when children and families are identified, following assessment, to have more complex needs. Multiple-professional and multi-agency involvement is essential in order to mediate risk.

All practitioners in health and social care need to be aware of their roles and responsibilities as well as the roles and responsibilities of others, including families, individual practitioners and organisations.

Capacity of nursing and midwifery practitioners

Along with contemporary child care policy a plethora of supporting documents published across the four home nations explicitly state standards of expected practice of all practitioners within universal services in order to meet policy outcomes. Competency frameworks are often used as the benchmark, stating the defined behaviours as well as expected and required outcomes to fulfil a specific task. In the case of nurses, midwives and other healthcare practitioners, the National Health Service (NHS) introduced a Knowledge and Skills Framework (KSF) (Department of Health 2004). The framework of defined competencies specifies levels of knowledge and skills required for each defined post-holder within health-care organisations. This is a generic framework, which explicitly identifies the required competencies, consisting of knowledge, skills and behaviours, relating to core as well as to specific domains of practice.

More specific competency frameworks designed to meet the standards of care in the provision of children and family services have been developed and integrated into the NHS KSF. One example is the *Core Competency Framework for the Protection of Children* (NHS Education for Scotland 2011). A further example was published by the Royal College of Paediatrics and Child Health in 2010, entitled *Safeguarding Children and Young People: Roles and Competences for Health Care Staff*. This framework is an intercollegiate document developed by a large number of disciplines representing nurses, midwives and a number of medical specialist services.

While competency frameworks have a number of strengths in preparing the healthcare workforce, there is one significant issue that must be addressed. Much of the literature defining competencies uses terms such as 'knowledge', 'skills', 'attitudes' and 'traits', to name but a few. Yet there is very little acknowledge-ment of the emotional content of competencies. There is now a growing evidence base which has identified that emotional competencies contribute to our health and well-being in, some would suggest, a significant way. Emotional intelligence which underpins emotional competencies also has a growing evidence base when it comes to decision making. Yet, neither emotional competencies nor emotional intelligence appear to be worth noting when considering the preparation of nurs-ing and midwifery practitioners. Further research into the effectiveness of com-petency frameworks and their part in the preparation of nurses and midwives in response to the safeguarding agenda is required.

Reflective activity

Reflecting on your own practice, consider how prepared you are to address the universal needs of children in your present clinical placement.

Can you identify what further knowledge and skills you will require to work with children and their families?

EMERGING THEMES

Legislation and contemporary child welfare policies have done much to support the place of children and young people in society. However, there are concerns that the present and far-reaching economic and social policies will not support the broader requirements of safeguarding children, young people and their families. The on-going evidence acknowledging the level of child poverty would suggest that for some children the risks imposed by disadvantage will continue to impact on their welfare and development. This indicates that their human rights, as well as the rights of childhood, are at risk of being denied. Further research is required to assess the unmet as well as the met needs of children and young people in the United Kingdom.

The educational and developmental preparation of nursing and midwifery practitioners to engage in child safeguarding practices needs to be addressed in full. There is insufficient research to ascertain whether practitioners delivering universal services are effective in their role to meet the needs of children and their families. While the preparation of practitioners has been identified as a priority in a number of government documents, there is a lack of transparency as to how health boards have prepared qualified nursing and midwifery practitioners to work with children and families.

Related to the preparation of nursing and midwifery practitioners is the use of competency frameworks in practice. While such frameworks are commonly used in healthcare education, there is little evidence that specific areas, such as emotional competencies or indeed emotional intelligence, are considered. Yet, there is evidence which suggests that these elements are important when it comes to practice. The emotional influences in decision making in child safeguarding are rarely addressed, thereby leaving a significant gap in our understanding of practice at the point of delivery.

CONCLUSION

This chapter has provided a brief historical review of the development of social welfare policy impacting on child welfare in the United Kingdom. Influential factors such as the rights-based agenda, legislative environment and evidenced-based interventions were discussed.

In response to the evolving political environment, public health was identified as the way to deliver changing policies. Questions around the preparedness of all practitioners to fulfil their roles and responsibilities in relation to the child welfare agenda were asked. The use of knowledge and skills frameworks was set out, but their efficacy was questioned. In particular, the lack of transparency regarding the impact of emotional competencies or indeed emotional intelligence was highlighted and questioned. A number of challenges remain as practitioners appear to be resistant to changing practice despite a raised awareness.

While children and young people have become a focus of policy, and practice development is supported by conventions and legislation, the reality may be more complex. These complexities are explored further in the following chapters.

FURTHER READING

Barlow, J. and R. Calam (2011) A public health approach to safeguarding in the 21st century. *Child Abuse Review* 20: 238–255.

Blackie, J. and Patrick, H. (2001) Medical treatment. In E. Sutherland and A. Cleland (ed.), *Children's Rights in Scotland*, 2nd edn. Edinburgh: W. Green/Sweet and Maxwell.

Brewer, M., J. Browne, Joyce, R. and Sibieta, L. (2010) *Child Poverty in the UK Since 1998/99: Lessons from the Past Decade*. IFS Working Paper. London: Institute for Fiscal Studies.

Evans, D. (2003) New directions in tackling inequalities in health. In J. Orme, J. Powell, P. Taylor and M. Grey (eds), *Public Health for the 21st Century*. Maidenhead: Open University Press.

Hall, S. (2011). The march of the neoliberals. *The Guardian*, 12 September.

Lindsey, D. (1994) *The Welfare of Children*. New York: Oxford University Press.

Northern Ireland Assembly (1995) *The Children (Northern Ireland) Order*. London: Secretary of State.

O'Donnell, M., Scott, D. and Stanley, F. (2008) Child abuse and neglect – is it time for a public health approach? *Australia and New Zealand Public Health Journal* 32: 325–330.

REFERENCES

Acheson, D. (1998) *Independent Inquiry into Inequalities in Health*. London: Directorate of Public Health.

Allen, G. (2011) *Early Intervention: The Next Step: An Independent Report to Her Majesty's Government*. London: The Cabinet Office.

Baker, M. (2011) Universal early childhood interventions: What is the evidence base? *Canadian Journal of Economics* 44(4): 1069–1105.

Beveridge, W. (1942) *Social Insurance and Allied Services*. London: HMSO.

Centre for Excellence and Outcomes in Children and Young People's Services (C4EO) (2011) *Grasping The Nettle: Early Intervention for Children, Families and Communities*. London: Social Care and Institute for Excellence.

Cunningham, J. and Cunningham, S. (2012) *Social Policy and Social Work*. London: Learning Matters.

Department for Education (1989) *The Children Act*. London: HMSO.

Department for Education (2013) *Working Together to Safeguard Children: A Guide to Inter-agency Working to Safeguard and Promote the Welfare of Children*. London: The Stationery Office.

Department for Education and Skills (2003) *Every Child Matters*. London: The Stationery Office.

Department for Education and Skills (2004) *The Children Act*. London: HMSO.

Department of Health (2004) *The NHS Knowledge and Skills Framework (NHS KSF) and the Development Review Process*. London: Crown.

European Court of Human Rights (1950) *European Convention on Human Rights*. Strasbourg: European Court of Human Rights.

Foley, P., Roche, J. and Tucker, S. (eds) (2001) *Children in Society: Contemporary Theory, Policy and Practice*. New York: Palgrave in association with The Open University.

Frieden, T. (2010) A framework for public health action. *American Journal of Public Health* 100(4): 590–595.

Henricson, C., and Bainham, A. (2005) *The Child and Family Policy Divide: Tensions, Convergence and Rights*. York: Joseph Rowntree Foundation. Available at: www.jrf.org. uk/sites/files/jrf/1859353312.pdf (accessed 31 January 2012).

HM Government (1998) *The Human Rights Act*. London: HMSO.

Kelly, M. (2003) Foreword. In J. Orme., P. Taylor, T. Harrison, M. Grey (eds), *Public Health for the 21st Century*. Maidenhead: Open University Press, p.xiv.

Kennedy, I. (2001) *Learning from Bristol: The Report of the Public Inquiry into Children's Heart Surgery at the Bristol Royal Infirmary 1984–1995*. London: The Stationery Office.

Laming, Lord (2003) *The Victoria Climbié Inquiry*. London: HMSO.

Lowden, J. (2002) Children's rights: A decade of dispute. *Journal of Advanced Nursing* 37(1): 100–107.

Marshall, G. (1998) *Oxford Dictionary of Sociology*. Oxford: Oxford University Press.

Miller, C. (2003) Public health meets modernisation. In J. Orme, J. Powell, P. Taylor and M. Grey (eds), *Public Health for the 21st Century*. Maidenhead: Open University Press. pp. 31–47.

Munro, E. (2011) *The Munro Review of Child Protection: Final Report. A Child-centred System*. London: Department of Education.

NHS Education for Scotland (2011) *Core Competency Framework for the Protection of Children*. Edinburgh: NHS Education for Scotland.

NSPCC (2011) *Child Abuse and Neglect in the UK Today*. London: NSPCC.

Roberts, M. (2001) Child care policy. In P. Foley, J. Roche and S. Tucker (eds), *Children in Society; Contemporary Theory Policy and Practice*. New York: Palgrave in association with the Open University. pp.52–64.

Royal College of Paediatrics and Child Health (2010) *Safeguarding Children and Young People: Roles and Competences for Health Care Staff*. Intercollegiate Document. London: Royal College of Paediatrics and Child Health.

Scally, G. (2003) Public health: a vision for the future. In J. Orme, J. Powell, P. Taylor and M. Grey (eds), *Public Health for the 21st Century*. Maidenhead: Open University Press. pp. 48–56.

Scottish Executive (2001) *For Scotland's Children: Better Integrated Services*. Edinburgh: The Stationery Office.

Scottish Executive (2002) *It's Everyone's Job to Make Sure I'm Alright: Report of the Child Protection Audit and Review*. Edinburgh: Scottish Executive.

Scottish Executive (2005) *Getting it Right for Every Child: Proposals for Action*. Edinburgh: Scottish Executive.

Social Exclusion Unit (1998) *Bringing Britain Together: A National Strategy for Neighbourhood Renewal*, Cm 4045. London: The Stationery Office.

Social Exclusion Unit (2001) *A New Commitment to Neighbourhood Renewal: National Strategy Action Plan*. London: Cabinet Office.

Social Services Inspectorate (2006) *Our Children and Young People – Our Shared Responsibility: The Reform Implementation Process in Child Protection Services in Northern Ireland*. Belfast: Department of Health, Social Services and Public Safety.

Spicker, P. (2008) *Social Policy: Themes and Approaches*. Bristol: Policy Press.

United Nations (1989) *United Nations Convention on the Rights of the Child*. Geneva: United Nations.

Vincent, S. (2010) An overview of safeguarding and protecting children across the UK. In A. Stafford, S. Vincent and N. Parton (eds), *Child Protection Reform Across the United Kingdom*. Edinburgh: Dunedin Academic.

Vincent, S. and Daniel, B. (2010) Where now for 'child protection' in Scotland? *Child Abuse Review* 19: 438–456.

Welsh Assembly Government (2004) *Children and Young People: Rights to Action*. Cardiff: Welsh Assembly Government.

2

KEY THEMES IN SAFEGUARDING AND PROTECTING CHILDREN AND YOUNG PEOPLE

SANDRA RODWELL AND GILL WATSON

CHAPTER SUMMARY

For many children living in the United Kingdom, the family environment is sufficient and wholesome enough, providing the ingredients to support their sequential development across physical, social and psychological domains. 'Sufficient and wholesome' in this context refers to the quality of parental sensitivity demonstrated through emotional warmth and timely and developmentally appropriate interaction by parents towards their children. For some children, however, the qualities of parental sensitivity are limited or insufficient, impacting negatively on a child's developmental potential, contributing towards child maltreatment. Anecdotal stories heard through media accounts and reported inquiries into child deaths highlight the fact that for some children, family life can be toxic. There are occasions when children are harmed outwith the family environment. The abduction and probable murder of April Jones in 2012 (Morris 2013) is just one representation of such a case.

AIM OF THIS CHAPTER

The overall aim of this chapter is to introduce the key concept of child abuse and neglect and factors which have the potential to impact on the response of healthcare practitioners. This chapter lays the foundation for the wide-ranging discussions running through this book.

Learning outcomes

After reading this chapter and following a period of reflection the reader will be able to:

- Define child abuse and neglect.
- Critically review the extent to which child abuse and neglect take place in the lives of children and young people.
- Identify the factors at the level of the individual and the organisation which may impact on the response of practitioners in their everyday practice.

Key terms

child abuse and neglect; incidence and prevalence rates; rights of the child

CHILD ABUSE AND NEGLECT IN THE LIVES OF CHILDREN

It is most likely that there are multiple inter-related factors, conditions and relationships contributing towards the significant harm experienced by children and young people, such as parental physical and mental ill-health, environmental conditions and childhood characteristics. While poverty and socioeconomic disadvantage have often been identified as a cause, not all parents living in low-income families abuse or neglect their children. While poverty is associated with the stress of meeting the needs of a family on low income, there is no direct evidence to confirm that poverty causes parents to maltreat their children (Dyson 2008). What is known is that becoming a parent can be a taxing and emotionally difficult time and not always the joyful event most often spoken about. Where parents more frequently report their parenting experience as emotionally stressful, the sensitivity required by parents to care for their children can be inhibited, possibly leading to the risk of harm.

However, it is not only within the home that children and young people may be exposed to significant harm. Some of our treasured and trusted institutions within the United Kingdom have also failed to protect children and in some cases have been reluctant to admit to, and address, past abuses. It is, however, more recent revelations which have had a profound impact within British society and have probably done more to raise awareness of just how vulnerable children and young people can be. In January 2013, the Metropolitan Police Service, along with the NSPCC, published their findings of Operation Yew Tree, an investigation into the many allegations of sexual abuse made against Jimmy Savile. The report, entitled *Giving Victims a Voice* (Gray and Watt 2013), is a factual account of numerous reports of sexual abuse carried out by Jimmy Savile spanning 54 years. At the time of publication 214 criminal offences were officially recorded, with further victims to be interviewed. While the majority were children, adults were not excluded from the reported cases of abuse by Savile. Many of the premises where Savile is alleged to have abused his victims are places where vulnerable people are cared for, such as hospitals and schools, as well as a hospice. The premises of the British Broadcasting Company (BBC) also proved to be unsafe for young people, as Savile allegedly abused some of his young followers within what has generally been considered a respected broadcasting institution.

DEFINING CHILD ABUSE AND NEGLECT

Many definitions of what constitutes child abuse and neglect have been developed and used to identify the extent of the problem. The International Society for the Prevention of Child Abuse and Neglect (ISPCAN) compared definitions from a total of 58 countries across the world and identified a number of common elements. However, one area that has proven to be problematic is the emphasis placed on the focus of the definitions. For example, should definitions focus on adult behaviour towards children, or impact/outcome of abuse towards children? This raises a number of issues as well as highlighting a number of gaps. If definitions focus on adult behaviours, does this include patterns of practices from national, educational, legal and health institutions which may contribute to the commission of bad practices or omission of appropriate care? If on the other hand the focus of definition was child outcomes of abusive care, should we then define what was intended abuse or indeed unintended? Such arguments have prevented an overarching definition of child maltreatment until the World Health Organization (WHO) developed what appears to be a definition focusing on the impact, potential or actual, of maltreatment towards the child by an individual or institution. What perhaps makes this definition more acceptable is that it is framed around the United Nations Convention on the Rights of the Child (1989).

The WHO developed what could be considered an encompassing and comprehensive definition, stating that:

> Child abuse or maltreatment constitutes all forms of physical and/or emotional ill-treatment, sexual abuse, neglect or negligent treatment or commercial or other exploitation, resulting in actual or potential harm to the child's health, survival, development or dignity in the context of a relationship of responsibility, trust or power. (2007: 8)

Table 2.1 Subtypes of maltreatment

Subtype	Definition	Added comments
Physical abuse	Any intentional use of physical action against a child that causes or is likely to cause harm to the child's health, survival, development or dignity, including beating, kicking, shaking, biting, strangulation, scalding, burning, deliberate poisoning and suffocation, or failure to prevent physical injury (or suffering) (WHO 2007).	Physical abuse includes hitting, shaking, throwing, poisoning, burning or scalding, drowning, suffocating, or otherwise causing physical harm to a child. Physical harm may also involve fabrication of illness by a parent or other which may lead to treatment that can harm the child (Browne et al. 2007).
Sexual abuse	The involvement of a child in sexual activity, either by adults or by other children in a position of responsibility, trust or power over the child, that the child does not fully comprehend, is unable to give informed consent to or is not developmentally prepared for, or that violates the laws or social taboos of society (WHO 2007).	Sexual abuse includes forcing or encouraging a child or young person to participate in sexual activities, including prostitution. This includes both physical (including sexual penetration using vagina, anal or oral sex) and non-physical acts including exposing sexual parts (flashing), forcing children to look at sexual imagery (e.g. pornography) or touch sexual organs or facilitating a child to behave in other sexually inappropriate ways (Department of Health 2006).
Emotional and psychological abuse	Any isolated action or pattern of failure over time on the part of a parent or caregiver to provide a developmentally appropriate and supportive environment. Abuse of this type includes: restriction of movement; patterns of belittling, blaming, threatening, frightening, discriminating against or ridiculing; and other non-physical forms of rejection or hostile treatment that has the potential to damage the child's physical, mental, spiritual, moral or social development. All abuse involves some emotional maltreatment (including witnessing the abuse of others) (WHO 2007).	Emotional or psychological abuse involves persistent and/or intermittent emotional maltreatment of a child. It can involve behaving towards a child in a way that makes them feel worthless, unloved or inadequate. Also behaving towards a child that leaves them isolated from others. Blaming, intimidating and terrorising a child, making them feel in danger. Witnessing violence towards another person may also cause psychological abuse. Any form of child abuse can lead to psychological abuse (Department of Health 2006).

Subtype	Definition	Added comments
Neglect	Failure on the part of a parent or other family member to meet the physical and/or psychological needs of the child through inadequate care or failure to protect the child from exposure to danger, either during isolated incidents or as a pattern of failure over time. Neglect can be associated with one or more of the following: health, education, emotional development, nutrition, shelter and safe living conditions (WHO 2007).	Neglect is the persistent or intermittent failure to attend to the child's developmental needs, including health; education; safe living environment; emotional support and a lack of support from others for physical and mental health needs; moral and spiritual needs. This definition also includes lack of effort to supervise and guide as much as is possible to do so (Browne et al. 2007).
Exposure to intimate partner violence	Witnessing behaviours that are actual or threatening towards another individual of a physical, emotional or psychological, or sexual nature by a current or former partner or spouse among heterosexual or same-sex couples even without sexual intimacy (Centers for Disease Control and Prevention 2010).	Exposure to intimate partner violence involves any form of violence towards another in the home. Hearing about violence can inflict harm, but witnessing violence against another may lead to violent behaviour in adulthood. Children can experience a number of emotional problems from anxiety, acute stress and post-traumatic stress disorder (Hamby et al. 2011).

For operational purposes, the WHO (2007) states that abuse and neglect needs to be further defined into four subtypes:

- Physical abuse
- Sexual abuse
- Psychological abuse (sometimes referred to as emotional abuse)
- Neglect

Table 2.1 presents definitions for the most common subtypes of maltreatment.

In more recent years witnessing intimate partner violence is now accepted as a further subtype of abuse (Gilbert et al. 2009).

It is important to highlight that experiencing one type of harm does not exclude other forms of abuse from occurring in tandem. However, experiencing any form of abuse or neglect can impact negatively on psychological well-being and future development (Hart and Glaser 2011).

A further point for all practitioners to consider is that the United Kingdom is populated by people from diverse cultures. To put it another way, the United Kingdom is a nation of multi-cultural people with differing rituals, values and beliefs regarding children and young people. While many cultures hold respectful beliefs, some rituals, for example female reproductive mutilation or under-aged organised marriages, are not tolerated within United Kingdom legislation or culture and have no value in our society.

Finally, the United Kingdom has become home, and a place of refuge, for families who have managed to escape from war-torn countries. Many have experienced a number of traumas caused by any number of abuses. It is therefore important for practitioners to be aware of such possibilities when caring for children and families from countries experiencing violence and other atrocities.

WHAT IS THE EVIDENCE?

The collection of official statistics relating to child maltreatment contributes, in part at least, to the repository of evidence which underpins policy development within the United Kingdom. Gathering data on the incidence as well as the occurrence of child maltreatment provides one strand of important evidence.

There is a substantial difference between reporting of child maltreatment to child protection agencies and the actual occurrence of abuse and neglect. This is recognised as problematic not only within the United Kingdom but also across the United States of America, Australia and Canada (Gilbert et al. 2009). The imbalance between occurrence and reporting of child maltreatment is of major concern, leading many to consider that what is recognised through reporting is actually only the 'tip of the iceberg'. A further concern is that data collected over the last five years suggests that the number of reported cases of child maltreatment continues to rise in all the four home nations.

INCIDENCE

National data sets recording the number of children placed on the child protection register or who are subject to a child protection plan are recorded annually across all four nations. Table 2.2 presents data collected from 2007–2011.

From the United Kingdom perspective there has been an obvious increase in the incidence of children being placed on either the child protection register or subject to a child protection plan each year. When each home nation is considered individually, however, there is a differing trend, with the reported number of cases from Scotland and Northern Ireland halting between 2008 and 2010, whereas both England and Wales demonstrated an on-going rise in the number of cases reported across the five-year period.

Reflective activity

Reflecting on the presentation in Table 2.2, consider the following questions:

- Does the rising trend of reporting result from an actual increase in the number of children being maltreated?
- Can we be sure that the increasing trend of reporting captures *all* children who are maltreated?
- What part does increasing awareness of health, education and law enforcement professionals play in the rise of reported cases?
- Are there reasons for the differences between and across the four home nations?

Table 2.2 Number of children on child protection registers or subject to a child protection plan on 31 March 2011

Nations	2007	2008	2009	2010	2011
England [1]	27,900	29,200	34,100	39,100	42,700
Scotland [2]	2,593	2433	2,682	2,518	2,571
Wales [3]	2,325	2,320	2,510	2,730	2,880
Northern Ireland [4]	1,805	2,071	2488	2,361	2,401
United Kingdom	34,623	36,024	41,780	46,709	50,552

1. **England:** Department for Education (2011), available online at www.education.gov.uk/rsgateway/ DB/STR/d001041/index.shtml
2. **Scotland:** Scottish Government (2012), available online at www.scotland.gov.uk/ Publications/2012/02/7586/downloads#res-1
3. **Wales:** Welsh Assembly Government (2011), available online at www.statswales.wales.gov.uk
4. **Northern Ireland:** Waugh, I. and Fitzpatrick, M. (2012), available online at www.dhsspsni.gov.uk/ children_order_trends_2011_-_tabbfinal.pdf

PREVALENCE

While it is important to understand the incidence of children recorded on the child protection register or subjects of a child protection plan, this data does not identify the actual number of children or adults within the population who have been exposed to abuse and or neglect. This specific information is known as the prevalence. Prevalence can only be identified through robust research studies governed by ethical principles and the use of specific research designs. Specific methods of sampling, sample sizes and data collection facilitate the calculation of an estimated percentage of the population of children and young people who have been maltreated. Such methods enable the findings to be generalised to the larger population.

However, in more recent years research studies using specific designs have been used. Such studies use retrospective methods of data collection by asking adolescents in differing age groups about their childhood experiences. Longitudinal studies of this nature are rare; however, two studies using a retrospective random probability design gathered data using the same questions posed to adolescents and parents. These studies provided evidence of prevalence across time (Cawson et al. 2000; Radford et al. 2011). When comparing Cawson et al.'s (2000) study and the more recent research by Radford et al. (2011), there is a reduction in reported prevalence of maltreatment in 18–24-year-old young people. While this outcome is positive, Radford and colleagues go on to acknowledge that:

> There is still a substantial minority of children and young people today who are severely maltreated and experiencing abuse at home, in school and in the community, from adults and from peers.
>
> Almost 1 in 5 11–17s (18.6%), 1 in 4 18–24s (25.3%) and 1 in 17 (5.9%) under 11s had experienced severe maltreatment during childhood. (2011: 118)

RISK FACTORS

Identifying occurrence and prevalence rates, though helpful, does not distinguish the environmental conditions in which abuse occurs. Messages emerging from research draw attention to the structural, economic and bio-psycho-social complexities and their relationships which underpin and maintain child abuse and neglectful events. In general terms, the greater the socioeconomic disadvantage experienced by a child and a family correlates with greater morbidity and premature mortality. Likewise, children living in disadvantaged households are at greater risk of experiencing adversity, incorporating poor developmental opportunities, poor family relationships, family conflict and at times violence. While some families are resilient to socioeconomic adversity, others are less able to overcome the stresses of parenting their children under such conditions (Wilkinson and Pickett 2010).

The evidence from research and reviews highlights that rarely is just one risk factor to blame for maltreatment. More frequently multiple risk factors are the cause, with socioeconomic conditions appearing as the strongest risk factor which is more likely to inhibit parental capacity (NSPCC 2011; Vincent and Petch 2012; Cuthbert et al. 2013). Further risk factors are found in communities with minimal resources to support the needs of families (Sidebotham et al. 2006).

From the perspective of the child much depends on the developmental stage and again parental capacity. Infants under one year of age are at increasing risk of harm because of their developmental immaturity. Parents who have little or no experience of caring for a newborn infant require guidance from family, friends and practitioners. However, infants living with a parent experiencing domestic violence, using substances or with a problematic mental health concern are at greater risk of significant harm (Cuthbert et al. 2013).

Reflective activity

Consider the role of the practitioner in identifying those at risk of harm.

SAFEGUARDING CHILDREN

The narrow approach of past child protection policies has failed to address in full the significant harm which some children experience. Therefore it is no wonder that policies within the United Kingdom, as well as in other developed countries, are moving away from the narrowly focused child protection policies of the past to adopt a population-based approach where the underlying principle is that all children and young people are potentially at risk of harm.

The move from narrow child protection policies to the much wider approach referred to as child safeguarding has at times been difficult for some to grasp. The lack of transparency as to where the term 'safeguarding' originated and how it is defined has not helped. For clarity on this point we must look to Article 19 of the 1989 United Nations Convention on the Rights of the Child (UNCRC) which states that:

> Children have the right to be protected from being hurt and mistreated, physically or mentally. Governments should ensure that children are properly cared for and protect them from violence, abuse and neglect by their parents, or anyone else who looks after them. (Article 19: Protection from all forms of violence)

Article 19 is explicit in stating that children should be secure and safe from harm. Governments have a responsibility to ensure that they are safeguarded from those who may harm them. The term 'safeguarding' to the intent of Article 19 therefore implies the actions of keeping a child secure and safe from harm. For the purpose of this book, safeguarding children and young people involves placing the child or young person at the centre of decision making, respecting their rights, demonstrated by the provision of the developmentally appropriate care required to achieve a level of wellness in both their physical and mental health while proving protection from emotional, physical and social obstacles in order to achieve well-being.

THE ROLE OF PRACTITIONERS

Practitioners within healthcare are in an ideal position to safeguard children and young people. Preparing and supporting parents to provide developmentally appropriate and sensitive care is possibly the most significant early intervention for reducing the threshold of risk and facilitating resilience. Equally, the same practitioners are also in a position to identify those children and young people who are at risk of experiencing harm.

While contemporary child care policies and the accompanying guidance to support changes in healthcare practice have been available for some years, recent evidence suggests that not all practitioners are prepared or equipped to take on their new roles and responsibilities.

A review of serious case reviews in England identified areas of concerns relating to interagency professional working and training and education of professionals (Brandon et al. 2011). Further, Gilbert et al. (2009) state that health professionals, including nurses and midwives, have in the past been slow to respond to child protection issues, citing lack of knowledge and inability to develop working relationships with families and other professionals. More recently, the attitudes and behaviours of nurses regarding reporting of child abuse and neglect have been explored (Piltz and Wachtel 2010) across a number of developed countries. The reported findings highlight a major barrier to nurses reporting abuse and neglect of children: lack of education. Nurses were reported as having limited experience in the area of child protection; poor documentation systems; fear of the consequences of reporting; and a lack of available emotional support following involvement in child protection work.

Less is known about midwives' earlier perspectives of the need to consider the rights of the newborn. However, it is not unreasonable to consider that a midwife's relationship with a mother and infant in her care is shaped by her beliefs of how motherhood is socially constructed (Chapman 2002). There is a danger, therefore, that for some individual midwives motherhood is solely viewed as a time of nurturing the newborn infant, when in fact it can be a time of vulnerability for the mother, induced by earlier social, psychological and economic hardship. Such beliefs, supported by a lack of insight into the impact of vulnerabilities, may indeed lead to a lack of recognition of an infant at risk of harm. This means that nursing and perhaps midwifery practitioners may enter clinical practice without the correct level of development and preparation. This in turn has consequences for undergraduate nursing and midwifery education programmes and all practitioners currently delivering services in adult, child, mental health and learning disability fields of nursing and midwifery. Good practice guidelines and standards suggest that all practitioners should be equipped with the required knowledge, analytical and relational communication skills necessary for safeguarding children. At the same time they should be able to recognise thresholds of risk and danger and report such findings to the appropriate agency, in line with local safeguarding policies. Being aware of 'what to do next' requires an understanding of the processes inherent in their clinical area. What are the steps to follow if, or when, suspicion of maltreatment arises? Finally, effective regular robust supervision is required with those qualified to carry out this important role and not just left to the underskilled line manager.

EMERGING THEMES

It is not possible to identify accurately the number of children and young people who have experienced or are experiencing exposure to harm.

Social welfare policies in the United Kingdom are responding to the child-centred approach to care, and healthcare practitioners are well situated to identify and report cases of suspected child maltreatment. However, lack of knowledge, skills and emotional support can impact negatively on their ability to respond.

CONCLUSION

This chapter has explored the context of child maltreatment within the United Kingdom. While much of the reported cases of significant harm of children and young people have been instigated by parents, there is also evidence to suggest that children and young people remain at risk of harm from outwith the family environment. Some of the most popular institutions in British society have been found to cover up past harms towards children and young people.

A definition of child maltreatment was provided, along with a description of the most common sub-types of maltreatment reported in the United Kingdom. The incidence and prevalence of child maltreatment was identified which provides some idea of the extent of the problem. However, it was also recognised that the identified number of reports may only represent the 'tip of the iceberg'.

Finally, evidence was presented which illuminated that the nursing workforce may not be prepared to fulfil the roles to address child safeguarding. Certainly, there was evidence that in some situations, nurses were unable to take responsibility for identifying and reporting harm towards children.

FURTHER READING

Cuthbert, C., Rayns, G., Stanley, K. (2013) *All Babies Count: Prevention and Protection for Vulnerable Babies*. London: NSPCC. Available at: www.nspcc.org.uk/inform/resourcesfor-professionals/underones/all_babies_count_pdf_wdf85569.pdf (accessed 20 December 2013).

Hamby, S., Finkelhor, D., Turner, H. and Ormrod, R. (2011) Children's exposure to intimate partner violence and other family violence. *Juvenile Justice Bulletin*. Office of Justice Programs, Office of Juvenile Justice and Delinquency Prevention, US Department of Justice. pp. 1–12. Available at: www.ncjrs.gov/pdffiles/ojjdp/232272 (accessed September 2013).

World Health Organization (2007) *Preventing Child Maltreatment in Europe: A Public Health Approach*. Copenhagen: WHO Violence and Injury Prevention Programme. Available at: www. euro.who.int/__data/assets/pdf_file/0012/98778/E90618.pdf (accessed 20 December 2013).

World Health Organization (2010) Child maltreatment: Fact sheet No. 150. Available at: www.who.int/mediacentre/factsheets/fs150/en/index.html (accessed 20 December 2013).

REFERENCES

Brandon, M., Sidebotham, P., Bailey, S. and Belderson, P. (2011) *A Study of Recommendations Arising from Serious Case Reviews 2009–2010*. Norwich and Coventry: University of East Anglia and University of Warwick.

Browne, K., Hamilton-Giachritsis, C. and Vettor, S. (2007) *Preventing Child Abuse in Europe: A Public Health Approach Policy Briefing*. Rome: WHO Violence and Injury Prevention Programme.

Cawson, P., Wattam, C., Booker, S. and Kelly, G. (2000) *Child Maltreatment in the United Kingdom: A Study of the Prevalence of Child Abuse and Neglect*. London: NSPCC.

Centers for Disease Control and Prevention (2010) *Injury Prevention and Control. Intimate Partner Violence: Definitions*. Atlanta, GA: CDCP. Available at: www.cdc.gov/ violenceprevention/intimatepartnerviolence/definitions.html (accessed October 2013).

Chapman, T. (2002) Safeguarding the welfare of children: 1. *British Journal of Midwifery* 10(9): 569–572.

Cuthbert, C., Rayns, G. and Stanley, K. (2013) *All Babies Count: Prevention and Protection for Vulnerable Babies*. London: NCPCC.

Department for Education (2011) Characteristics of Children in Need in England: Financial Year 2010 to 2011 – Final Figures. London: Crown. Available at: www.education.gov.uk/ rsgateway/DB/STR/d001041/index.shtml (accessed 20 December 2013).

Department of Health (2006) *Working Together to Safeguard Children*. London: Department of Health.

Dyson, C. (2008) *Child Protection Research Briefing: Poverty and Child Maltreatment*. London: NSPCC.

Gilbert, R., Spatz Widom, C., Browne, K., Fergusson, D., Webb, E. and Janson, S. (2009) Burden and consequences of child maltreatment in high-income countries. *Lancet* 373: 68–81.

Gray, D. and Watt, P. (2013) *Giving Victims a Voice: Joint Report on Sexual Allegations Made Against Jimmy Savile*. London: Metropolitan Police Service and National Society for the Prevention of Cruelty to Children. p. 39.

Hamby, S., Finkelhor, D., Turner, H. and Ormrod, R. (2011) Children's exposure to intimate partner violence and other family violence. *Juvenile Justice Bulletin*. Office of Justice Programs, Office of Juvenile Justice and Delinquency Prevention, US Department of Justice. pp. 1–12. Available at: www.ncjrs.gov/pdffiles/ojjdp/232272 (accessed September 2013).

World Health Organization (2007) *Preventing Child Maltreatment in Europe: A Public Health Approach*. Copenhagen: WHO Violence and Injury Prevention Programme. Available at: www.euro.who.int/__data/assets/pdf_file/0012/98778/E90618.pdf (accessed 20 December 2013).

Hart, S. and D. Glaser (2011) Psychological maltreatment – maltreatment of the mind: a catalyst for advancing child protection toward proactive primary prevention and promotion of personal well-being. *Child Abuse and Neglect* 35: 758–766.

Morris, S. (2013) April Jones murder: how detectives pieced together her final hours. *The Guardian*, 30 May. Available at: www.theguardian.com/uk/2013/may/30/april-jones-murder-final-hours (accessed October 2013).

NSPCC (2011) *An Analysis of Serious Case Reviews Concerning Children Under One*. London: NSPCC.

Piltz, A. and Wachtel, T. (2010) Barriers that inhibit nurses reporting suspected cases of child abuse and neglect. *Australian Journal of Advanced Nursing* 26(3).

Radford, L., Corral, S., Bradley, C., Fisher, H., Bassett, C., Howat, N. and Collishaw, S. (2011) *Child Abuse and Neglect in the UK Today*. London: NSPCC.

Scottish Government (2012) Children's Social Work Statistics Scotland, No.1. Edinburgh: Crown. Available at: www.scotland.gov.uk/Publications/2012/02/7586/downloads#res-1 (accessed 20 December 2013).

Sidebotham, P. and the ALSPAC Study Team (2006) Patterns of child abuse in early childhood: a cohort study of the 'children of the nineties'. *Child Abuse Review* 9311–9320.

United Nations (1989) *United Nations Convention on the Rights of the Child*. Geneva: United Nations.

Vincent, S. and Petch, A. (2012) *Audit and Analysis of Significant Case Reviews*. Wolverhampton and Edinburgh: University of Wolverhampton/Institute for Research and Innovation in Social Science and the Scottish Government.

Waugh, I. and Fitzpatrick, M. (2011) *Children Order Statistical Trends for Northern Ireland 2005/06 to 2010/11*. Belfast: Information and Analysis Directorate. Available at: www.dhsspsni.gov.uk/children_order_trends_2011_-_tabbfinal.pdf (accessed 20 December 2013).

Welsh Assembly Government (2011) *Children on Child Protection Register by Local Authority, Category of Abuse and Age Group*. Cardiff: StatsWales. Available at: https://statswales. wales.gov.uk/Catalogue/Health-and-Social-Care/Social-Services/Childrens-Services/ Service-Provision/ChildrenOnChildProtectionRegister-by-LocalAuthority-PeriodOfTime (accessed 20 December 2013)

Wilkinson, R. and K. Pickett (2010) *The Spirit Level: Why Equality is Better for Everyone*. London: Penguin.

World Health Organization (2007) *Preventing Child Maltreatment in Europe: A Public Health Approach Policy Briefing*. Available at: www.euro.who.int/__data/assets/pdf_file/0012/98778/E90618.pdf (accessed October 2013).

3

ATTACHMENT

GILL WATSON AND LYNN KELLY

CHAPTER SUMMARY

Over the last three decades there has been a surge of interest across professional disciplines into the emerging research exploring infant brain development and the impact of the early evolving attachment relationships between infants and parents. Infant brain development and the formation of attachment relationships should not be viewed as separate entities, or coincidental in nature, but rather as a significant partnership which impacts on the changing architecture of the infant brain across infancy, childhood, adolescence into adulthood.

An attachment relationship is special because it has a number of important qualities which differentiate it from other types of relationships. First, it is the initial social relationship an infant will experience with other humans. It is this relationship that lays the foundations for the development of all future relationships. Second, the attachment is developed to the parents who experience proximity to and interaction with the infant. Third, becoming attached involves the development of an attachment bond which endures over long periods of time (Cassidy 1999). The quality of this developing relationship has a significant influence on infants' physical, social and emotional development, including their evolving personality.

Attachment relations founded on parental sensitivity towards meeting their infant or young child's needs support that child to reach their potential. However, those infants and young children exposed to parents less sensitive to their needs because of substance misuse or violence face a future that might include periods of depression or self-destructive behaviours (van der Kolk 2005).

New advances in technologies, including magnetic resonance imaging (MRI), have identified the significant impact attachment relationships have on the first three years of the developing brain mediating the young child's mental health, including emotional, social and personality outcomes (Thompson 2000). There is now a significant evidence base to suggest that the quality of the early attachment a young child develops with their parents provides the foundation for their subsequent physical and emotional development and behaviours (Perry 1994).

Practitioners working, either directly or indirectly, with children and their families must have knowledge and understanding of the influence that the infant–parent relationship has on the subsequent development of infants and young children. Such knowledge and understanding informs the very practices we use, to engage, support and provide realistic and applicable interventions to support infants, young children and their families.

This chapter will explore the development and significance of attachment relationships between infants and parents. A description of how attachment forms and the properties which contribute to its development is provided. Parenting behaviours are described and their significance on the infant's ability to experience sequential developmental milestones is discussed. A table integrating parenting behaviours and infant sequential development over the first three years is presented. Finally, the chapter concludes with a description of infant neurological development within the context of the infant–parent attachment relationship.

AIMS OF THIS CHAPTER

This chapter has two aims. The first is to identify and examine attachment relationships and the impact parental caregiving behaviours can have on infant neurological development and functionality. The second aim is to explore attachment through the lens of developmental trauma.

Learning outcomes

After reading this chapter and following a period of reflection the reader will be able to:

- Describe the main concepts of attachment and the environmental properties known to influence the quality of the relationship.
- Identify and discuss the significance of parental behaviours on infant and child development taking into account the psycho-social and economic conditions which influence parental caregiving.
- Identify and discuss how the quality of attachment can impact on all aspects of child development, with specific attention and emphasis on emotional regulation and social integration.
- Consider how healthcare practices can support or hinder facilitation of early attachment relationships between infants and their parents.

Key words

attachment relationship; infant mental health; insecure attachment; neurological development; secure attachment; sensitive parenting behaviours; trauma

ATTACHMENT

Social interactions are simply the means by which we develop, grow and continue to learn throughout our lifetime (Pridham et al. 2009). Such interactions are powerful mechanisms influencing the way we learn to think (cognitions), feel (emotions) and behave (act). The manner in which we learn to interact with others is mediated by a number of ecological elements, such as the culture and social groups we belong to, as well as the economic and physical and psychological environment in which we live (Hinde 1997). However, one of the most significant influences on our ability to interact with others is the first relationships we develop following birth. More often than not the first social interaction experienced by infants is with parents or primary care givers. It is the quality of this first relationship that lays the foundations for social interactions with others throughout the years in our life-span. In this chapter we will refer to parents and primary care givers as 'parents' for ease of reading, but it is important to remember that the primary care giver need not be a birth parent.

The parent's relationship to their infant is called a 'caregiving' relationship, as they carry out caregiving behaviours through their caring and interactive role. While parents are generally the main caregivers, in the absence of parents, others can and do fulfil this role. Infants and young children are capable of developing multiple attachments. This is common when there are siblings and grandparents who interact with the infant in some capacity on a regular basis. It is not uncommon for there to be a hierarchy of attachment figures with the infant or young child selecting the person who best meets their needs at the time of distress (Cassidy 1999). The differing styles of interaction are what contribute to the individual differences within and across attachment relationships. For example, parents can often interact with one child, yet use a different style of interaction with another child in the same family. This is because although every attachment and caregiving relationship experiences similar processes, they each have an individual pattern of interaction which is unique to that specific relationship.

THEORIES SUPPORTING THE NEED FOR ATTACHMENT AND CAREGIVING RELATIONSHIPS

There are a number of theoretical explanations which support the need for attachment relationships. Three of the more common are protection, supporting child development and emotional regulation, and finally a combination of both. The theory of protection is underpinned by evolutionary theory, whereby protection becomes a strategy to enable an individual to survive through infancy into adulthood. On reaching adulthood the person is then able to reproduce to maintain the survival and continuity of the human genome. An alternative perspective is that attachment supports child development from infancy onwards. This is required because when compared to other mammals, human infants are the most immature and take much longer to develop into adulthood; however, they have a greater ability to learn. A third perspective involves the integration of protection to support child development, in particular infant neurological development.

In more recent years neurological development in infancy and childhood has received much attention because it is now recognised that the first three years of a young child's life is the time when major neurological pathways develop, such as those influencing emotional and social regulation. The psycho-social interactive attachment and caregiving experiences between the infant and parent mediate how these pathways evolve, impacting on cognitive and personality development, adaptability, as well as how well a child learns to self-regulate their own emotions and behaviours when interacting with others (Perry et al. 1995). The first three years of a child's life and the environment in which they live, mediated through their parents, is significant in shaping their ability to develop in later years.

PARENTING (CAREGIVING) BEHAVIOUR

Parents have a very important role to play in the lives of their children. A central concept in the development of a caregiving relationship is the ability of parents to respond sensitively to their infant's developmental needs. While there is every reason to consider that both mothers and fathers are capable of being sensitive to their infant and young child's needs, by far the majority of evidence has been gathered from the mother's perspective with the exclusion of fathers. While there is a growing evidence base exploring fathers' perspective in this area, no definition of parental sensitivity can be identified. Shin et al.'s definition of maternal sensitivity is used to support understanding of sensitive parenting behaviour:

> [M]aternal sensitivity is the quality of a mother's sensitive behaviours that are based on her abilities to perceive and interpret her infant's cues and respond to them. A mother's sensitive behaviours must be contingent on her infant's prior to behaviours and reciprocal with her infant. It is a dynamic process which accompanies the adaptation and changeability. (2008: 307)

This definition identifies the importance of maternal behaviour towards their infant. What is important is the ability of mothers to react appropriately within the best timeframe to meet their infant's needs. To be sensitive, according to Shin et al. (2008) mothers need to be perceptive to their infant's developmental ability and needs; interpret their infant's cues; and be able to respond appropriately. Before mothers learn to respond appropriately to their infant's cues they require cognitive and psychological abilities to engage with their infant, viewing their infant as the central character in their lives. It is the mother's ability to master the necessary behaviours facilitated through being emotionally available to perceive, interpret and respond appropriately within the correct timeframe. It is these attributes that contribute to reciprocal and timely interaction between the mother and her infant. Not all mothers have the necessary skills when first becoming a parent. Some parents will take longer to develop the necessary skills and expertise. Much will depend on their prior experience.

Reflective activity

From your experiences and knowledge, take a few minutes to consider how new parents develop the necessary knowledge and skills to understand their new infant's needs.

As the infant develops beyond their first year, maternal behaviour changes for two significant reasons. First, as the infant develops into their second year of life, their needs change. Second, maternal perceptions and interpretation of their infant's cues alter as they become more experienced is assessing the needs of their infant (Shin et al. 2008).

Although Shin et al. (2008) focused on maternal sensitivities and behaviours, there is no evidence to suggest that fathers are unable to display the same caregiving behaviours and sensitivities.

THE INFLUENCE OF CAREGIVING BEHAVIOUR ON THE SECURITY OF INFANT/CHILD ATTACHMENT

The quality of an infant's attachment relationship to their parents has a significant impact on their development. Patterns of sensitive parenting behaviours are more likely to facilitate what is termed a secure attachment relationship before the end of the infant's first year (National Scientific Council on the Developing Child 2007). With sensitive parenting, infants learn that their emotional, along with their physical and social needs, will be met. In this environment, the transition from infancy to early childhood supports development of social and cognitive skills, but most importantly children learn to regulate their own emotions (Bowlby 1998). This in turn enables the child to develop more positive coping skills (Feeney 2000) and at the same time build resilience and protective skills into an organised strategy to manage challenging events in childhood and beyond. Overall, the infant and subsequent child who experiences secure attachments with their parents are more likely to achieve better educational, health, including mental health, and social relationship outcomes when compared to those children who experience insecure attachment relationships with their parents.

Insecure attachments are more common in infants and young children exposed to less sensitive patterns of care from their parents over a protracted period of time. The relationship is marked by varying inconsistent and inappropriately responsive social interactions. Infants and young children may be deprived in some degree from appropriate developmental physical, psychological and social sensitive stimulation. Such adverse parenting behaviours contribute towards poorer health and social outcomes (Feeney 2000) and emotional distress (Schore and Schore 2008), leading to poor psychological coping strategies (Glaser 2000). These all increase the risk of infants and young children experiencing failure-to-thrive through neglect (Drotar and Robinson 1999), contributing to developmental delay (Perry et al. 1995; To et al. 2001; Moutquin 2003), post-traumatic stress syndrome, anxiety states and depression (Perry 1994; Perry et al. 1995; Schore 2001a, 2001b). Similar outcomes and behaviours are also experienced by older children and adolescents, impacting on poor educational attainment, truancy, illegal behaviours and drug and alcohol problems. Many go on to experience difficulties in forming relationships with others with an increased risk of experiencing a reduced quality of life (National Scientific Council on the Developing Child 2010).

The quantity and quality of inappropriate parenting interaction can lead to three possible attachment outcomes. The first two involve the child developing a strategy for coping with and responding to inappropriate parenting styles; that is, either insecure avoidant or insecure ambivalent parenting styles (Prior and Glaser 2006). The third possible outcome is that the child will not have a strategy that sufficiently manages inappropriate parental responses and interactions. This is a more likely outcome when parents appear an object of fear, leading the child to experience conflict and uncertainty demonstrated by a disorganised way of attempting to manage or cope with situations (Prior and Glaser 2006). A child who develops an insecure disorganised attachment to their parents is more likely to experience poor long-term outcomes across all domains; for example, emotional regulation, social interactions, academic outcomes and behaviour problems (Prior and Glaser 2006).

CONDITIONS INFLUENCING PARENTAL ABILITY TO DEVELOP SENSITIVE CAREGIVING BEHAVIOURS

What has become clear is that all infant-to-parent attachments are different. This is because the psychological and social contextual conditions in which every attachment relationship develops are different (Weinfield et al. 1999). This is evident in practice when infant–parent relationships develop at differing paces, and parental behaviours and interaction with their children are viewed as being quite different. This is very acceptable and should not be viewed with suspicion. Parents and infants/children develop a level of synchrony pertinent to their own and unique interactive relationship.

Psycho-social conditions impact on many factors in the infant–parent environment. Proximal conditions involve the characteristics of the infant, such as infant

Table 3.1   Conditions impacting on parental responsiveness to infant

Previous attachments are important. Early attachment experiences influence our ability to interact with others. The environment in which an infant develops an attachment to their parents is strongly influenced by intergenerational behaviours. Parents who had a secure attachment to their own parents are more likely to be sensitive and responsive with their own infants while parents who experienced a more dismissive relationship with their parents are more likely to behave in the same way towards their infants. However, regardless of a parent's own childhood attachment experiences, their ability to reflect and discuss their early experiences in a coherent manner suggests that they are more autonomous in their own parenting behaviours and emotions.

Acceptance of the pregnancy and the fetus is a process in itself, often punctuated by events throughout the pregnancy. For example, confirmation of the pregnancy, images from ultrasonic investigations, quickening and physical changes accompanying the maturing pregnancy. Such experiences, though often associated with maternal–fetal attachment, are equally experienced by prospective fathers. The meaning of these experiences needs to be considered in relation to how both parents feel about the pregnancy. Unplanned pregnancies do not always mean unwanted; however, the circumstances leading to the pregnancy itself may interfere with the acceptance of the pregnancy and fetus.

A favourable environment to support the development of attachment involves interaction between physical, emotional and social elements of the environment. Belsky (1999) identifies the many proximal elements influencing attachment security. However, he also identifies the importance of more distal elements of the psycho-social environment and their impact on the developing attachment. Relationships between parents, the level and quality of social support and the wider social world influence the context in which all family relationships develop. It is reasonable therefore to consider the impact that the early home environment can have on a developing attachment between infant and parent.

Physical and emotional availability of parents is an essential prerequisite to the development of parental responsiveness and sensitivity, especially in the first year of the infant's life. Such qualities are considered a prerequisite to the development of a secure attachment. Being able to perceive, accurately interpret and respond appropriately to their infant's behaviour and emotions is the hallmark of sensitive parenting. Parents who experience stress, mental ill-health, including depression and substance misuse, can be at greater risk of not interacting on an emotional level with their infant. Equally, parents who have experienced abuse in their own childhood can be overly intrusive towards their infants. Other situational factors, for example maternal ill-health or geographical reasons, may contribute to a lack of physical availability.

Parental sensitivity is a technical term that defines a set of focused, empathic and communicative skills which enable parents *to perceive*, *accurately interpret* and *respond appropriately* to their infant's behaviours. Parents who are sensitive move beyond merely recognising the physical and emotional needs of the infant. By viewing the world from their infant's perspective as well as 'reading' and learning by observing their infant's early behavioural cues, parents are more able to understand and respond to their infant's needs. Parental sensitivity is a major component in the development of a secure attachment relationship between infant and parent.

temperament, appearance and health (Shin et al. 2006; Shin et al. 2008). Other proximal conditions relate to the characteristics of the parents, for example: previous attachment experiences; impact of intergenerational attachment experiences (Belsky 1999); level of education; their psychological and mental health; and relationship dysfunction, such as intimate partner violence and quality of social support (Weinfield et al. 1999). This list is not exhaustive. More distal conditions involve the level of community cohesion, the physical environment, quality of amenities, quality of health services and socioeconomic status. To summarise, there is not one single factor responsible for influencing parenting behaviour but a combination and interaction of multiple factors both proximal and distal within the overall parental environment. Some of the main proximal and distal conditions which are recognised as impacting on parental caring behaviours are described in Table 3.1.

Reflective activity

Reflecting on the contents of Table 3.1, can you identify the distal and proximal conditions impacting on parental responsiveness to their infants?

PROTECTION, RISK, RESILIENCE AND ADAPTATION

Conditions that are favourable and positive are more likely to facilitate parental behaviours which best support the formation of secure infant–parent attachments. A secure attachment supports timely and appropriate infant and child development across the early years. These conditions are considered protective in nature and more likely to result in the developing child adapting well to changes within their environment. When conditions are less favourable, resulting in fewer protective factors, there is an increased likelihood of risk to the developing infant-to-parent attachment and subsequent infant and child development. In these circumstances children can be at risk of developing insecure attachments to their parents, rendering them less likely to adapt to changes in their environment. However, regardless of the level of risk factors, their impact may change as the individual infant/child develops (Masten and Gewirtz 2008). This potential outcome highlights two points: first, attachment security can change over childhood; and second, not all attachments exposed to greater risk and vulnerability result in insecure attachments and associated developmental concerns (Weinfield et al. 1999; Masten and Gewirtz 2008).

Reflective activity

Why do some families manage risk and vulnerabilities more favourably than others?

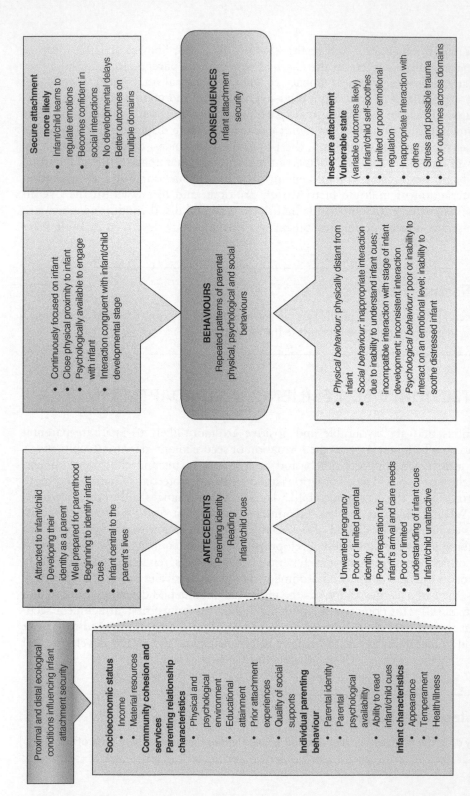

Figure 3.1 Determinants influencing parental physical, social and psychological behaviours impacting on infant attachment security

Figure 3.1 is a framework providing the antecedents, behavioural conditions and consequences of parental physical, social and psychological behaviours which are recognised as impacting on infant attachment security.

The following case study represents a situation recognised by many practitioners working in practice today. Working with uncertainty and complexity is the most challenging aspect of professional practice. This point is highlighted and discussed in detail in Chapter 4. The often complex nature of family life and its inherent and intertwined relationships does not pose easy answers for the practitioners. This case study provides the practitioner with the opportunity to consider and apply their theoretical understanding of attachment relationships and how the quality of the attachment can inform the assessment process. Based on a synthesis of the assessment findings, interventions can then be identified and targeted towards keeping the child safe and at the centre of the decision making process.

Jennifer is an 18-year-old single mother who gave birth to her daughter 3 months ago. The birth was straightforward but the child, Donna, was born at 36 weeks weighing 2000 grams. The pregnancy was unplanned; however, Jennifer decided to keep the baby and appears to love the child. Jennifer smokes cigarettes and although she tried to stop during her pregnancy she admitted to having started again. Donna's father is the long-term partner of Jennifer but his current whereabouts are not known. The parents have a chaotic relationship marked with occasional drug and alcohol use. When drinking, they can often be violent towards each other.

Jennifer was 6 years old when she was taken into the care of the local authority. She had been living with her mother up until this point but was removed at the request of her mother who was experiencing a severe and enduring episode of depression. Jennifer's mother died less than one year later, and the cause of her death was never established. Jennifer had a grandmother who remained in contact with her and occasionally had her to stay for short periods, but this never became a permanent arrangement due to the grandmother's ill-health.

Up until the age of 10 years Jennifer experienced several changes of foster parents. These changes in her placement were due to foster carers moving on or changes to her care plan which meant that she was not assessed as in need of a permanent carer until she was 10 years old. When Jennifer was 10 years old she was eventually placed with long-term foster carers on a permanent care order and remained with this family until she left home at 16 years of age. Jennifer was offered a place in an independent living unit providing support to young people to live independently. Jennifer moved into her own council flat when she was 17 and had been managing her day-to-day responsibilities. She was also beginning to consider doing a short course at the local college when she found out that she was pregnant. Jennifer remains in regular contact with her foster parents who are very supportive of her and her baby.

The health visitor has been visiting Donna and Jennifer since they arrived home from hospital. The foster mother is usually at home with Jennifer when she visits and seems to carry out many of the routine tasks for the baby such as feeding and changing.

(Continued)

(Continued)

Jennifer has resumed smoking but claims that she no longer drinks alcohol or takes drugs. Jennifer has a lot of friends and there are often several young people in her flat for long periods of time. The health visitor has a good relationship with Jennifer and believes that the physical care of the child is being met; however, she is concerned that the emotional needs of the baby are not being attended to adequately.

If you were the health visitor what information would you require to ensure that Donna was safe and that all of her physical, social and emotional needs were being met? Refer to Figure 3.1 while considering the following questions:

- What factors reassure you that Donna is well cared for?
- What are the factors you consider to be the most concerning?
- Considering the factors identified in response to the last question; what evidence would you need to have before feeling confident that the risks could be managed safely?
- Can you identify the additional support that Donna might need?
- Can you identify who would be best placed to provide this?
- What factors would you look out for to indicate that the situation has deteriorated and that the child might now be at significant risk?
- What would you do if the risks to Donna were to increase?

INTEGRATION OF INFANT/CHILD DEVELOPMENT AND PARENTAL CAREGIVING BEHAVIOURS OVER THE FIRST THREE YEARS

The purpose of this chapter was to examine the significance of attachment and the attachment relationships infants develop to their parents and how this relationship shapes the developing brain in the first three years of life. In Table 3.2 we provide a timetable of interaction accounting for the integration of infant development and functional capabilities with parental behaviours. The intention is that this information can help to guide your understanding of what is broadly termed normal developmental interaction for both infant and parent. We reiterate that this is a timetable of expectation and must not be viewed as a rigid account of what should happen. Remember every attachment between infants and their parents is heterogenic, with each process moving forward at its own pace but within a broad timeline.

As highlighted earlier, one of the main purposes of attachment relationships is to support child development. This is managed through the unique and interactive experiences between infant and parent whereby repeated patterns of play and learning build the architecture of the developing infant brain (see Table 3.2).

Table 3.2 Integration of infant development and functional capabilities with parental behaviours

Timing of development	Infant	Parent (attachment figure)
Phase 1 ***After birth*** *(following an uncomplicated delivery)*	• Normal biochemical changes resulting from the birthing process lead to the infant being in a wakeful state and ready to interact with others after birth. • Infant is unable to discriminate between individuals, therefore does not have a preference as to whom they may interact with (Prior and Glaser 2006). • Within the first days the infant has developed a preference for their mother's breast milk. • Infant starts to imitate parental behaviours after immediate viewing, e.g. facial expressions, figure and arm movements.	• In most cases parents are ready to interact with their infant. This is a time of introductions, exploration and orientation through close proximity. • For mothers the release of oxytocin, a neuropeptide, at the time of birth leads to a reduction in anxiety and a rise in emotional warmth, often displayed towards the infant. • Should breast-feeding be initiated at this time, further maternal oxytocin is released. • Physical interaction between fathers and their infants can raise paternal oxytocin levels.
After 2 days *of proximity and interaction*	• Infant also starts to recognise the faces of those they have interacted with using mechanisms such as direct gaze recognition. • Full face exposure to parents helps the infant to recognise and discriminate parental features.	• Parents start to discriminate the characteristics and behaviours of their own infant, recognising their infant's non-verbal behavioural cues very quickly in the first few days. • Parents want to be in close proximity to their infant. • The infant is a central feature in the lives of parents.
Phase 2 ***Within 2–4 months***	• The first months are a time of developmental change, in particular auditory and visual sensory ability. • Infant becomes more responsive to parents, learning to read parental cues. • Infant begins to develop an expectation of how each parent will behave in future interactions. • Infant can imitate facial expressions up to 24 hours after viewing them. Indication of implicit memory (cognitive) development.	• Parents spend more time interacting with their infant. • Mutual eye gazing starts to develop, which frequently includes verbal exchanges, often with each partner taking turns. • Intuitive parenting usually starts now as parents adjust their communicative interactions with their infant to meet their infant's developmental abilities.

(Continued)

Table 3.2 (Continued)

Timing of development	Infant	Parent (attachment figure)
Phase 3 *Within 5–7 months*	• Infant's physical development on-going; now able to turn to view other activities within the environment. • Infant's cognitive development can be viewed through implicit (procedural) memory demonstrated by fine motor and perceptual skills. • Infant's emotional development demonstrated by their awareness of their own subjectivity, a level of awareness of their own emotions. • This level of (primary) subjectivity leads to infant demonstrating goal-directed behaviour to gain proximity to parents when feeling under threat or stressed. • Infant's goal-directed behaviour involves infant signalling their perception of something threatening or stressful to their parents through crying or raising arms towards parent.	• Sensitive parenting responses to their infant are crucial at this time. • Sensitive parenting requires parents to be able to perceive, interpret and respond appropriately to their infant's signals. • Parental ability to be empathic towards their infant, viewing the world from their infant's perspective. • Parental behaviours towards their infant need to accommodate the infant's evolving developmental and specifically emotional abilities. • Parents need to respond to their infant's emotional negativity, learning to soothe their infant's stress. • The level of sensitivity demonstrated by parents can have a significant positive impact on the quality of the developing attachment relationship between infant and parents.
Within 9–12 months	• Infant continues to develop a strong preference for one or more attachment figures (parents). • The security of the attachment provides protection and comfort while enabling independent exploration within the environment. This is aided by the infant's physical development, e.g. crawling and walking. • Infant learns to communicate their emotions through nonverbal and verbal sounds. • Emotions generally expressed through need, e.g. feeling hungry, cold or hot.	• Parental sensitivity remains an important feature at this time. However, parents also need to develop awareness that their infant is an independent psychological agent' Meins (1997) refers to this realisation as mind-mindedness, which involves a realisation of their infant's mental state. • The development of attunement between infant and parent continues. A patterned relationship evolves as infant and parent become increasingly familiar with each other's behaviours, responses and rhythms when interacting. • Parents and infant communication and interaction evolves as parents leave longer gaps between responding to their infant's interactions in non-stressful encounters. The course and timescale of such changes is individualised within each infant–parent relationship.

Timing of development	Infant	Parent (attachment figure)
13–24 months (continuity and change)	• Infants continue to develop physically in growth and strength, impacting on mobility and reaching a stage of independent mobility.	• There develops more episodes of synchronised play between parent and infant.
	• Speech and language continue to develop, leading to the ability to use two or three words together by 24 months.	• Parents change their interactions in response to their infant's changing capacity.
	• Visual perceptual and fine motor skills become more sophisticated.	• Parents recognise their infant as an intentional agent now better prepared and developmentally ready to interact with a wider social world.
	• Socially, the infant and young child is content to play alone; prefers to be near a known adult; starts to exchange toys with other children.	• Parents let the infant explore but within the realms of a safe physical and social environment.
	• Cognitive development progresses with the formation of explicit memory, with auditory and visual recognition memory being the first explicit memory system to develop.	• Monitoring the infant exploring the environment is an important and necessary part of development.
		• Parent–infant communications remain important. Interactive conversations use narratives exposing the infant to past events and planning for the future.
	• With the development of language skills across year two, explicit memory becomes more sophisticated.	• Infant and young child introduced to and engaging with a wider social world.
	• Changes in emotional expression. Sympathy and empathy towards others.	
	• Emotional expression changing from expression of need to responses from experiences. Awareness that emotions of parents may be different from their emotions.	
	• Cognitions and emotions start to develop in tandem, regulated through the attachment relationship. This underpins the development of coping styles.	
Phase 4 25–36 months	• Towards the end of year two and into year three the attachment between young child and parent changes as the relationship enters this fourth and final phase. The young child becomes aware that the attachment figure has their set goals or motivations.	• By this phase of attachment continuity but also change feature. The young child and parent spend time apart, indicating that although physical closeness remains important, it is less intense.
	• The young child's physical, cognitive, social and emotional development is on-going as their social environment widens, involving the development of relationships with others.	• Parents maintain contact with the developing child through shared communication. Parent and child are drawn together more in 'partnership'.

The next section of this chapter provides a synopsis of infant neurological development before aligning this development to the evolving infant–parent attachment relationship. Infant development is a large area of study, therefore it is not possible to examine all developmental domains. In this chapter, we shall focus on the neurological processes which shape the brain architecture through the development of specific neural pathways, focusing on the domain of emotions.

INFANT NEUROLOGICAL DEVELOPMENT

The infant brain changes rapidly from pre-birth to the age of three years. At birth the term infant brain contains almost the adult quota of neurons. Connections between neurons are, however, very limited. The average infant brain weighs approximately 400 grams, rising to adult proportions at 1000 grams by 12 months of age (Glaser 2000). As the infant brain becomes more organised over the next 24 months, it appears similar in structure to the adult brain. With these changes, the architecture of the brain changes rapidly. By year three all major neuro-fibre tracks are present. As the neuro-fibres become operational, different parts of the brain connect to each other, enabling an increase in an infant and young child's functional capabilities. For example, within the first year there is an increase in visual acuity, as well as motor, cognitive, memory and behaviour skills (Parsons et al. 2010). Over the next two years, further changes in functional abilities continue to develop, especially in relation to memory and emotional regulation. Changes in the young child's behaviours, including the ability to mobilise, communicate with others as well as express their own needs, develop as a direct result from the structural and organisational changes which have taken place over the first three years of the child's life (Parsons et al. 2010).

Three basic processes guide the small cellular and larger regional changes which bring about alteration in the brain architecture over the first three years of development: genetics, experience-expectant and experience-dependent processes.

Genetics

Genetic processes influence development of the neural system from the first stage of neurogenesis to the final myelination process involving mature neurones and neural pathways. Gene expression follows a timetable of sequential events leading to the timely over-production of synapses and specific stages of development, referred to as critical or sensitive periods. However, if synapses are not used within a specific period, genetic processes cause unused synapses to be pruned back.

Experience-expectant processes

The second type of processes are called experience-expectant. These require parts of the brain to be genetically prepared, through the over-production of synapses to facilitate the necessary specific stimulus from the environment mediated by parents through infant–parent patterned interactions. The timing of this over-production of synapses is under the control of the genetic timetable. It is at this specific time, referred to as sensitive periods, when experiences created through infant–parent interaction result in the development of specific synapses.

Sensitive periods are important in the development of sensory nerve cells, such as auditory, visual and perceptual development. Should, for whatever reason, the stimulus from the patterned infant–parent interaction not reach the specific regions of the sensory brain within the sensitive period, then the neurones within the sensory regions are unlikely to develop fully or sufficiently well, impeding future development and potentially reducing functionality of the specific sensory organ. The unused synapses are then pruned back and once the critical or sensitive period for environmental stimulation has passed, underused synapses disappear. This outcome can have subsequent and serious consequences for future development of the specific pathway and other interrelated aspects of development. Such outcomes can arise for a number of medical or relationship issues which prevent the required sensory threshold being reached.

An example of the interaction between genetic and experience-expectant processes relate to the development of hearing and language development in the first and second years of life. Chronic or poorly treated ear infections in infancy can result in loss of hearing ability. Other problems in language development can arise when parents do not regularly and frequently interact with their infant, introducing new experiences through the use of language and other experiences.

Reflective activity

Reflecting on your understanding of the experience-expectant processes, can you identify what experiences or conditions have a positive and negative impact on the development of an infant's sensory organs?

Experience-dependent processes

The third aspect that impacts on infant and young child neurological development are those called experience-dependent processes. These specific processes result from the unique history of interactive experiences an infant or young child has with their immediate environment. The physical, social and psychological aspects of the infant's environment are generally under the control of parents. The rigid timetable of experience-expectant development is not relevant to experience-dependent processes. A further difference is that the synapses resulting from experience-dependent processes are found in regions of the brain which process information originating from experiential histories with others. Clearly, this is what makes us the individuals were are. It is the early experiences of infant–parent interaction through experience–dependent processes which shape the development of neural pathways that regulate physiological and emotional responses.

To summarise experience-dependent processes, parents who respond sensitively to their infants needs in a timely and appropriate manner support their infant's developing physiological and emotional neural pathways, enabling the developing infant and young child to adapt to changes in their environment and at the same time supporting the development of self-regulation. Conversely, parents who repeatedly display unresponsive, unpredictable or inappropriate behaviours can result in adverse developmental outcomes for their infant. The early stresses experienced by infants resulting from poor-quality parent interaction creates abnormalities within the neurotransmitter and neuro-hormonal systems which impact negatively on physiological and emotional developing neural pathways. Such an outcome can hinder future development of neurological structures primed to evolve in later stages of development (Perry 2009).

As highlighted earlier, there are a number of domains which develop across the childhood years into adulthood. These domains are all inter-related and impact on each other. However, the development of emotions and emotional regulation during infancy and childhood requires a special mention because of the influence this specific domain has on learning as well as cognitive and social competencies (Glaser 2000). What is striking is that a young child's emotional health is shaped by the emotional and social characteristics of the environment they have experienced (National Scientific Council on the Developing Child 2004). This point reminds us of the importance of the quality of infant-to-parent attachment.

THE DOMAIN OF EMOTION

Infants have limited control over their emotions. They do have the ability to communicate discomfort, such as hunger through crying. Ideally, parents respond appropriately, soothing the infant's distress. By two to three months infants' visual acuity has developed sufficiently for infants to recognise and share emotions through social interaction, synchronised eye contact and gazing (Parsons et al. 2010). The continuation of similar patterned interaction between infant and parent stimulates the formation of neural pathways between the early maturing right side of the brain and the limbic centres, which orchestrates emotions and the autonomic nervous system. The same neural pathways are responsible for activating physiological response to stress. According to Schore (2001a), it is the same neural pathways that lay down the foundation for an infant's mental health. Again, infants and young children who experience regular, patterned and appropriately sensitive interaction over time with their parents are more likely to experience optimal mental health characterised through their ability to be flexible and adaptable to changes in their environment. This infant and young child is more likely to gain greater confidence in regulating their emotions, using them to communicate appropriately to others their level of safety or indeed distress. This process takes time to develop as the young child reaches the age of three years.

Infants and young children exposed to patterns of inappropriate and less sensitive interactions across time are more likely to have difficulties regulating their own emotions and experience more stress. The resulting physiological outcomes can lead to poor ability to adapt to changes in their environment. It is this individual who is at increased risk of experiencing poor mental health as they evolve across the life span.

IMPACT OF STRESS AND MALTREATMENT ON THE DEVELOPING YOUNG BRAIN

For some infants and children exposure to maltreatment and stressful events can occur. Such events can be one-off or perhaps more frequent, such as exposure to physical abuse or sexual abuse. Other experiences are viewed as being more chronic in nature, such as neglect and or emotional abuse (Glaser 2000). Nevertheless, the impact on the young developing brain can be catastrophic. The threshold for harm may vary; however, there is growing evidence of a dose-related effect, with some children developing traumatic stress responses leading to post-traumatic stress disorder (PTSD) while others fail to experience stress in this way but development is nonetheless compromised. What is evident is that the outcome of exposure to stress or stress and maltreatment has an adverse impact on the developing brain (Belsky and de Naan 2010). The ability to recover can be mediated if the young child is supported by sensitive carers.

Infants as young as three months have presented a traumatic stress reaction following exposure to stressful events. The lack of a sensitive empathic parent leaves infants unable to process the emotions resulting from stressful interactions. The chronicity of inappropriate parenting behaviour impacts on the right side of the brain, influencing the neural pathways leading to the limbic area of the brain. Such experiences contribute to limitations in how the infant learns to regulate their emotions while at the same time increasing the autonomic nervous system activity. This increase in the autonomic activity leads to elevated levels of cortisol and other hormones which have an adverse impact on the developing brain, witnessed through infant and child behaviour and emotional responses such as continual crying; difficulty in being soothed; hyper arousal; problems with sleeping, eating, elimination; frustration; tantrums; and difficulty developing relationships (Lieberman 2004).

Chronic maltreatment events across the first three years interrupt the three basic processes which shape the architecture of the brain. Experience-expectant and dependent processes, if disrupted can over-ride genetic expression (National Scientific Council on

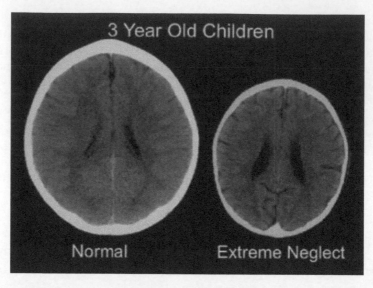

Figure 3.2 Two cerebral tomography scans (reproduced with kind permission from Kluwer Academic Publishers)

the Developing Child 2010). Likewise, neuro-developmental activities such as synaptogenesis and pruning, if also disrupted, can lead to a reduction in some or all areas of the brain, which reduces the functional capabilities of the young child. This outcome reduces cognitive, emotional and social development and capabilities. Figure 3.2 presents cerebral tomography scans of two 3-year-old-brains. On the left is the brain of a healthy 3-year-old child with an average head size (50th percentile). On the right is a brain from a series of three 3-year-old children who have experienced severe sensory deprivation neglect in early childhood. As can be seen, there is a significant difference between the two scans. The smaller of the two demonstrates abnormal development of the cortex (cortical atrophy) and other abnormalities suggesting abnormal development of the brain.

CASE STUDY

Six months on, Donna is still living at home with Jennifer. Her foster mother, Mrs Duncan, is still very much involved in the day-to-day care of Donna and now takes responsibility for most of Donna's care during the daytime. Jennifer is now going out with her friends on a regular basis, leaving Donna with Mrs Duncan. Donna's father has returned but has not shown any significant desire to be involved in Donna's life beyond making the occasional visit. The health visitor now has no concerns about Donna's physical care but is more concerned about the lack of interest and interaction between the mother and child. Jennifer is clearly very fond of her daughter but does not seem to understand how important their relationship is for Donna's long-term emotional security. Jennifer does not quite see the link between carrying out the routine tasks of feeding and settling her baby to sleep and the development of their relationship. Jennifer believes that as long as Donna is fed and cared for then she will be fine.

The health visitor is beginning to notice that Donna regularly looks to Mrs Duncan when Donna needs to be soothed and does not seem to engage with her mother in a similar way. Jennifer is also reporting that she is finding it difficult to settle Donna for bed and that she is now waking through the night and is not easily settled back to sleep. Jennifer is now finding that she is getting less sleep and is growing a little more agitated when she is talking about her child.

Again, imagine you are the health visitor caring for Donna and her mother, Jennifer. You have been learning about brain development and understand how important the first three years are for the healthy development of a child's brain. Consider now how you might use your knowledge of infant neurological development to work with Jennifer in order to assist her to better understand her attachment with her child. You may find Figure 3.2 helpful.

- It would be important for you to consider how the information about infant neurology is useful to supporting Jennifer and her child.
- Can you think of specific tasks and interventions you might suggest to help her become more attuned to the emotional needs of her child?

EMERGING THEME

The quality of the attachment relationship a child develops with their parents underpins such experiences. It is this relationship and the inherent patterned inter-actions which have a significant role in the infant and young child's neurological development and future physical, psychological and social domains.

Though not an emerging theme, this chapter has incorporated details of sensitive parenting to support practitioners develop awareness of its significance to the developing child in the first three years of its life.

CONCLUSION

The systematic physical, social and emotional processes inherent in the development of attachment relationships that infants and young children develop towards their parents and main caregivers has been discussed. The quality of parental sensitivity during the early years of development has been highlighted. The significance of such relationships in the sequential developmental process paying particular attention to the impact attachment and caregiving relationships have on infant neurological development has also been highlighted. Ecological elements in which family relationships evolve shape the individual differences in the formation of attachment relationships between an infant and the parents and other caregivers. While some parents have the ability to overcome risk and adversity through the provision of positive interpersonal interventions with their infant, other parents are less able to overcome similar difficulties. It is this latter group who are more likely to be less sensitive in their parenting capabilities. Such experiences can lead to a child developing an insecure attachment to their parents and can lead to a number of poor developmental outcomes. Some children can go on to experience significant trauma and morbidity.

FURTHER READING

Gerhardt, S. (2004) *Why Love Matters: How Affection Shapes a Baby's Brain*. London: Routledge.
Thompson, R. (2001) *Development in the First Years of Life: The Future of Children*. Princeton, NJ: Princeton Brookings. pp. 21–33.

REFERENCES

Belsky, J. (1999) Modern evolutionary theory and patterns of attachment. In J. Cassidy and P. Shiver (eds), *Handbook of Attachment: Theory, Research and Clinical Applications*. London: Guilford Press. pp. 141–161.
Belsky, J. and de Naan, M. (2010) Annual research review: parenting and children's brain development: the end of the beginning. *Journal of Child Psychology and Psychiatry* 52: 409–428.
Bowlby, J. (1998) *Attachment and Loss: Attachment*. London: Pimlico.
Cassidy, J. (1999) The nature of the child's ties. In J. Cassidy and P. Shiver (eds), *Handbook of Attachment*. London: Guilford Press. pp. 3–20.
Drotar, D. and Robinson, J. (1999) Researching failure to thrive: progress, problems and recommendations. In D. Kessler and P. Dawson (eds), *Failure to Thrive and Pediatric Undernutrition: A Transdisciplinary Approach*. Baltimore, MD: Brookes.
Feeney, J. (2000) Implications of attachment style for patterns of health and illness. *Child: Care, Health and Development* 26: 277–288.
Glaser, D. (2000) Child abuse and neglect and the brain – a review. *Journal of Child Psychology and Psychiatry* 41: 97–116.
Hinde, R. (1997) *Relationships: A Dialectical Perspective*. Guildford: Psychology Press.
Lieberman, A. (2004) Traumatic stress and quality of attachment: reality and internalization in disorders of infant mental health. *Infant Mental Health Journal* 25: 336–351.
Masten, A. and Gewirtz, A. (2008) Vulnerability and resilience in early child development. In K. McCartney and D. Phillips (eds), *Blackwell Handbook of Early Childhood Development*, vol. IV. London: Blackwell. pp. 22–43.
Meins, E. (1997) *Security of Attachment and the Social Development of Cognition*. Hove: Psychology Press.
Moutquin, J. (2003) Classification and heterogeneity of preterm birth. *BJOG* 110: 30–33.

National Scientific Council on the Developing Child (2004) *Children's Emotional Development is Built into the Architecture of their Brains.* Cambridge, MA: Harvard University Press.

National Scientific Council on the Developing Child (2007) *The Timing and Quality of Early Experiences Combine to Shape the Brain.* Working Paper No. 5. Cambridge, MA: Harvard University Press.

National Scientific Council on the Developing Child (2010) *Early Experiences Can Alter Gene Expression and Affect Long-term Development.* Cambridge, MA: Harvard University Press.

Parsons, C., Young, K., Murray, L., Stein, A. and Kringelbach, M. (2010) The functional neuroanatomy of the evolving parent–infant relationship. *Progress in Neurobiology* 91: 220–241.

Perry, B. (1994) Anxiety disorders. In C. Coffey and R. Brumback (eds), *Textbook of Pediatric Neuropsychiatry.* London: American Psychiatric Press.

Perry, B. (2009) Examing child maltreatment through a neurodevelopmental lens: clinical applications of the neurosequential model of therapeutics. *Journal of Loss and Trauma* 14: 240–255.

Perry, B., Pollard, R., Blakley, T., Baker, W. and Vigilante, D. (1995) Childhood trauma, the neurobiology of adaption, and 'use-dependent' development of the brain: how 'states' become 'traits'. *Infant Maternal Health Journal* 16: 271–290.

Pridham, K., Lutz, K., Anderson, L., Riesch, S. and Becker, P. (2009) Furthering the understanding of parent–child relationships: A nursing scholarship review series. Part 3: Interaction and parent–child relationship – assessment and intervention studies. *Journal for Specialists in Pediatric Nursing* 15: 33–61.

Prior, V. and Glaser, D. (2006) *Understanding Attachment and Attachment Disorders.* London: Jessica Kingsley.

Schore, A. (2001a) The effects of early relational trauma on right brain development, affect regulation, and infant mental health. *Infant Mental Health Journal* 22: 201–269.

Schore, A. (2001b) Dysregulation of the right brain: a fundamental mechanism of traumatic attachment and the psychopathogenesis of posttraumatic stress disorder. *Australian and New Zealand Journal of Psychiatry* 36: 9–30.

Schore, J. and Schore, A. (2008) Modern attachment theory: the central role of affect regulation in development and treatment. *Clinical Social Work Journal* 36: 9–20.

Shin, H., Park, Y. and Kim, M. (2006) Predictors of maternal sensitivity during the early postpartum period. *Journal of Advanced Nursing* 55: 425–434.

Shin, H., Park, Y., Ryu, H. and Seomun, G. (2008) Maternal sensitivity: a concept analysis. *Journal of Advanced Nursing* 64: 304–314.

Thompson, R. (2000) The legacy of early attachments. *Child Development* 71: 145–152.

To, T., Cadarette, S. and Liu, Y. (2001) Biological, social, and environmental correlates of preschool development. *Child: Care, Health and Development* 27: 187–200.

van der Kolk, B. (2005) Developmental trauma disorder: towards a rational diagnosis for children with complex trauma histories. *Psychiatric Annals* 35: 401–408.

Weinfield, N., Sroufe, L., Egeland, B. and Carlson, E. (1999) The nature of individual differences in infant–caregiver attachment. In J. Cassidy and P. Shiver (eds), *Handbook of Attachment: Theory, Research and Clinical Applications*, vol. 1. London: Guilford Press. pp. 68–88.

4

RISK ASSESSMENT

SANDRA RODWELL AND GILL WATSON

CHAPTER SUMMARY

The emphasis in nursing and midwifery practice is first to prevent significant harm from occurring, and second to identify the potential for harm as well as when harm has occurred. Assessing risk is a key public health intervention to safeguard and protect children and their families. Risk assessment begins before the birth of an infant and informs the core assessment which is routinely carried out after birth. This assessment is most often carried out by the family health visitor who is the named professional throughout the preschool years. The responsibility of the named professional is to co-ordinate a child's health and social care needs within a multi-professional environment. It is important that a child's perspective is articulated and heard.

Additional assessments will be required should parental capacity or other living conditions become compromised, thereby threatening the health and well-being of a child. Where there is on-going involvement of services, placement issues, or plans to reunite a child back with their family, an assessment of risk is required. On this occasion, social services take the lead, incorporating specialist assessments from the multi-professional team.

For nurses and midwives to participate in risk assessment and the wider risk management process, understanding of the underlying theories, activities and cognitive requirements are pivotal to the quality of decisions made throughout and at the end of the assessment process.

AIM OF THIS CHAPTER

The aim of this chapter is to explore the umbrella term 'risk management', with specific emphasis on the process of risk assessment as it is applied in the practice of child safeguarding. The quality of risk assessment structures and processes are discussed. A critique of role ambiguity and the resulting impact this can have on assessing risk within the context of multi-professional working is presented.

Learning outcomes

After reading this chapter and following a period of reflection the reader will be able to:

- Develop a better understanding of the need to assess risk in child safeguarding and protection.
- Reflect critically upon the different factors that contribute to the assessment of risk.
- Understand the purpose of a multi-professional contribution to the risk assessment process.
- Critically analyse the elements that impact on the quality of risk assessment.
- Begin to apply a critical approach towards professional decision making in risk management.

Key words

analysis; assessment framework; decision making; interventions; multi-professional; public health; risk assessment; synthesis

PUBLIC HEALTH AND CHILD MALTREATMENT

There has been an increase in the reporting of child maltreatment in recent years. This is possibly due to a number of reasons, such as increasing intolerance of child abuse and neglect in developed countries; greater awareness of child maltreatment by an increasing number of professional groups in health, education, law enforcement and the third sector, leading to increased reporting; and a change in policy direction (Gilbert et al. 2012). Failure to address the underlying issues allows ongoing suffering by many children from infancy to adolescence and beyond. Because child maltreatment is preventable, child safeguarding and protection are now viewed through a public health lens. Public health approaches to addressing preventable conditions such as child maltreatment (O'Donnell and Scott 2008) have proven successful when applied to other major health conditions resulting from unhealthy lifestyles such as smoking, drink-driving and poor diet.

Through the application of contemporary public health epidemiological methods, strategies to reduce the burden of child maltreatment within the United Kingdom are now in place. Such strategies have already gone some way towards informing child safeguarding policies which impact on everyday nursing and midwifery practice. Public health approaches are guided by a conceptual framework for assessment and provision of evidence-based interventions. Such an approach requires disciplined systematic activities to identify exposure and susceptibility, causation and pathways of causation within the developmental environment of every child which can contribute towards significant harm. This approach identifies vulnerabilities, referred to as risks, which increase the potential for harm under certain conditions.

RISK ASSESSMENT

Assessing risk identifies levels of exposure to harm in the population and the conditions which are recognised as contributing towards that risk. However, this becomes increasingly more difficult following patterns of long-term exposure under complex conditions (Grey and Sarangi 2003), which is often the case in child maltreatment. In such situations the assessment of any risk can appear less certain following analysis and synthesis of assessment data. Working with such levels of uncertainty has the potential to lead to the introduction of inappropriate interventions or no intervention at all. A further factor impacting on any assessment of risk is resilience, defined by Masten and Gewirtz as 'positive adaptation in the context of risk or vulnerability' (2009: 27).

Resilience, like risk, is conditional and dependent on exposure to conditions of risk. There needs to be evidence that regardless of this exposure to adversity, the individual is doing well and there are identified mediating factors.

Two theoretical approaches underpin the assessment and management of risk: the formation of infant–parent relationships (attachment theory) and the bio-psychosocial environment (ecological theory). These are interlinked.

THEORETICAL APPROACHES TO THE ASSESSMENT AND MANAGEMENT OF RISK

Attachment theory is the theory of child and relationship development between infants, children and their parents. Chapter 3 provides an account of attachment theory and the importance of the quality of sensitive parenting and the impact this has on the developing child. If parents are unable to respond sensitively in a consistent and timely manner over a significant period, their infant or child is at risk of significant harm.

A second theoretical approach used to frame risk assessment is that of ecological theory, which incorporates the developmental and environmental conditions. The

Table 4.1 The ecological environment (Bronfenbrenner 1979)

Level	Focus
Microsystem	The direct interaction between the individual and any one specific setting, e.g. the child and the family, however it is composed.
Mesosystem	Interaction between the different settings in which an individual is involved: the family; other relatives and friends; school; the wider community.
Exosystem	Factors in the wider social system in which the individual is embedded. The child is not directly involved but is affected by decisions made, such as parental employment; change in school resources. This level is influenced by local and national strategic decision making.
Macrosystem	Cultural values and beliefs which prevail within society, e.g. culture belief systems relating to the rights of the child; religious groupings; socioeconomic groups.

following section provides a brief explanation of ecological theory and its application to assessing risk.

Bronfenbrenner's (1979) seminal work was key to conceptualising an environment which was influenced by the characteristics of individuals, separately and together. Bronfenbrenner referred to the ecological environment as 'a set of nested structures, each inside the next, like a set of Russian dolls' (1979: 3). The ecological environment comprised four levels, as set out in Table 4.1.

The language adopted by Bronfenbrenner (1979) is not particularly accessible. Nonetheless, the values and principles inherent in the concept of an ecological environment which recognises the impact of the physical and social environment on behaviour has been widely adapted and adopted.

Building on the work of Bronfenbrenner (1979), Belsky (1993) applied a developmental ecological perspective to an exploration of the causal pathways to child abuse and neglect. Based on the premise that the circumstances which may result in child abuse and neglect are many and complex, Belsky focused his theoretical discussion around three 'contexts of maltreatment' (1993: 413). Each of the three contexts comprised a number of different aspects as set out in Table 4.2.

Table 4.2 Context of maltreatment (Belsky 1993)

Context	Different aspects
Developmental context	Factors specific to the parent, e.g. own childhood experiences; characteristics specific to the individual (personality, resources).
Immediate interactional context	Factors specific to the child, e.g. age; health; behaviour. Parenting and parent–child interactions.
Broader context	Community, cultural and evolutionary contexts.

The three contexts provided a framework within which Belsky (1993) interrogated the available evidence base specific to child maltreatment. The author found that within the evidence base there was little attempt to distinguish between child abuse and neglect. The findings presented by Belsky challenge the presumption that a specific set of circumstances will necessarily lead to child abuse and neglect. Central to the process of assessment which applies an ecological perspective is the concept of balance (Belsky 1993). A key principle stressed by Belsky is the need to take account of the balance between stressors and supports or risks and protective factors identified at the different levels. The ambiguity introduced through recognising the many factors which interact at different levels and circumstances opens up the opportunity for a more appropriate and flexible response to individual cases (Belsky 1993). Belsky concluded that the findings may be disappointing for those who would prefer a model which facilitates the development of a number of reliable predictive factors and associated solutions. However, this expectation is perhaps unrealistic.

While the appropriateness of dividing the social world into apparently arbitrary and discrete slices may be questioned, by applying the concept of an ecological environment to the process of assessing risk the ideological assumptions which shape the roles, responsibilities and actions adopted by individuals and organisations are rendered visible, highlighting the need for a multi-agency response.

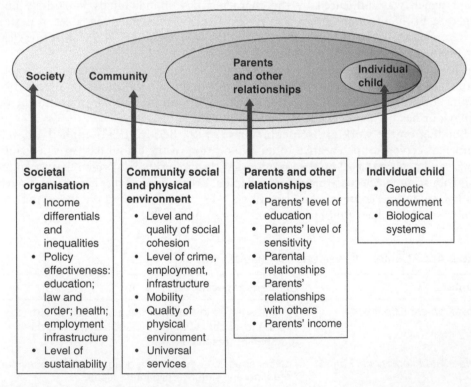

Figure 4.1 Ecological layers of influence

Drawing on the work of both Bronfenbrenner (1979) and Belsky (1993), Figure 4.1 provides an account of the factors to be considered in each of the layers of influence that interact with each other.

Attachment and ecological theories contribute towards a framework which enables a number of different factors to be considered. Practitioners' knowledge of the interaction between developmental and environmental factors underpins their ability to assess risk of exposure to potential or actual significant harm. While an assessment of risk can identify the potential for significant harm, there is a need to have a clear means of identifying exposure to actual significant harm. The defining characteristics of maltreatment and the different sub-types can make a substantial contribution to recognising the extreme level of risk a child can experience.

THE PROCESS OF RISK ASSESSMENT

There are common principles of agreement across all four home nations as to the structures underpinning the assessment framework (Horwath 2010). While each may be called by a different name, they all provide a comprehensive and ecological guide to assessment. Common to the assessment frameworks is a needs-led, evidence-based instrument designed to identify need in order that early interventions are introduced to prevent and reduce significant harm. These frameworks are no more

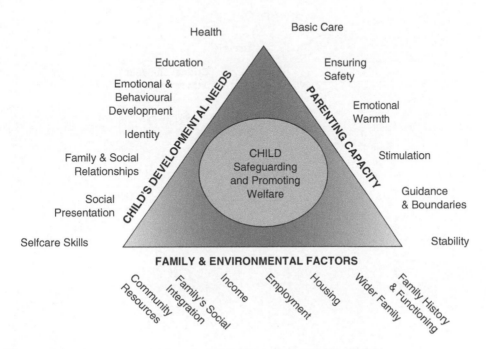

Figure 4.2 Assessment triangle (Department of Health 2000)

than a model which provides a structure to guide the assessment process. Structure is important especially when a situation appears complex. In such situations it is essential to be able to access all relevant information, concentrating on what is relevant. To be of value as well as rigorous, all aspects of the framework must be addressed in equal detail to allow a full and comprehensive understanding of the physical, social and emotional environment in which the child is developing. Figure 4.2 presents an example of the assessment triangle, commonly used within the United Kingdom. In the centre of the triangle, at the heart of the assessment process, sits the child whose needs are being assessed by considering their individual developmental needs, the capacity of their parents to provide the ideal physical, social and emotional environment, and the wider family and community resources needed to meet the child's developmental needs.

RISK ASSESSMENT IN PRACTICE

Assessment provides a means of identifying the unique characteristics of a child and the family environment in which that child develops. The framework and processes which guide assessment facilitate the recognition of vulnerabilities and valuable resources within the family environment. Identifying risk factors has a crucial role in planning tailored interventions best suited to address individual child and family

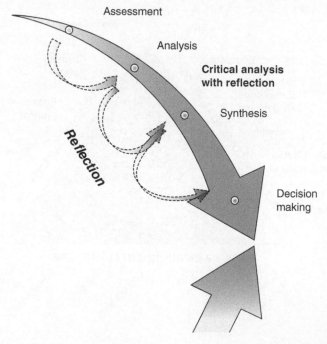

Figure 4.3   Risk management process

needs as well as contributing towards reviewing the effectiveness of such interventions (Horwath 2010). Within an ecological model, as well as working with individual families, educational interventions may be required to raise awareness of individual health and social care professionals, their organisations and the wider public.

The structures guiding the assessment – for example, the frameworks and tools as well as the processes, such as the style of communication and the ability to work in partnership with children, parents and the wider family and other professionals – impact on the quality of the overall risk management exercise. Understandably, it is the quality of the risk assessment that influences the other elements involved in managing risk, such as analysis, judgement and decision making. Figure 4.3 demonstrates the relationship between all the components of the risk management process, starting with risk assessment. Running in parallel with the process of risk management is reflection; a cognitive activity incorporating critical analysis. This will be discussed further under the section on professional practice below. The management of risk is an iterative process as more information is gathered.

MULTI-PROFESSIONAL ASPECTS IN RISK ASSESSMENT

The assessment of risk within a child's life is no longer the sole responsibility of one agency. Contemporary child welfare policy clearly specifies the contribution of all universal services and their practitioners (Munro 2011). Sidebotham and Weeks (2010) identify the need for involved services to change as a child moves from infancy into childhood and adolescence; for example health, followed by education services, remain the lead professions in the early years. This does not prevent other services supporting a child and family but may facilitate other services being involved. However, while this arrangement highlights the multi-professional approach, it does not identify the communication processes required when working across different professional groups, or the professional tensions that may exist.

The Victoria Climbié Report (Laming 2003) is just one of many reports about child deaths from abuse or neglect which are emphatic about the need for services to communicate and collaborate with each other more effectively and gain mutual respect in a trusting partnership. The most important aspects of this are the sharing of information with other agencies, appreciating the skills of other practitioners and being prepared to challenge when it is felt that a child continues to be at risk despite intervention. However, for a number of reasons this can prove challenging for individual practitioners from all services.

ROLE AMBIGUITY AND THE IMPACT ON MULTI-PROFESSIONAL WORKING

In response to the developing role for all healthcare workers in protecting children, as set out in *Protecting Children: A Shared Responsibility* (Scottish Executive

2000), Crisp and Lister (2004) interviewed nurses working in a community setting in one Scottish city. The aim of the exercise was to explore how nurses perceived their role and responsibilities in relation to protecting children. This was inclusive of nurses who did not work directly with children.

One of the key findings from this study was a degree of ambiguity among participants as to how the role of nurses in relation to child protection issues translates in practice. This lack of consensus was apparent in the responses of participants from the same discipline as well as between disciplines (Crisp and Lister 2004). Underlying the sense of ambiguity was a degree of tension generated by the expectations participants had of their own roles and the roles of others. The expectations placed on them by others also appeared to be an area of contention. For example, the authors found that some of the participants with health visiting experience considered their surveillance role as one which was imposed on them by social work colleagues and others within nursing. However, this role was seen to conflict with the main focus of their work providing support to vulnerable families. Health visitors also felt that not all nurses (for example, practice nurses) realised the potential that their own situation offered for child protection work, specifically in relation to education, support, identification and referral. Nonetheless, the authors note that participants other than health visitors and those working specifically with children also identified ways in which nurses could take a proactive role in relation to child protection concerns.

The authors concluded that there is a role for nurses working with adults in a community setting in relation to child protection. However, the extent to which nurses can work together to develop their child protection capacity requires further research. The authors made a number of recommendations focused at an organisational level. Key issues were the need for support for practitioners and recognition of the tensions they face when presented with seemingly competing agendas.

Although the sample was small in the study carried out by Crisp and Lister (2004), participants were selected for their ability to address the research questions. However, for a number of practical reasons midwives were not included. Neither were the interviews and focus groups recorded. While it was reported that extensive notes were taken, it may have been hard to capture all of the subtle nuances. It is also possible that the process of note-taking may have impacted on the flow of the discussions. However, even in situations where the role of nurses in relation to child protection is set out in law, a number of competing concerns may inform their decisions to report (Nayda 2002).

The study undertaken by Nayda (2002) was based on a small group of 10 registered nurses working in a community setting in Southern Australia where healthcare practitioners are legally bound to report cases of child maltreatment. While the participants were clear about their legal obligations to report their suspicions of child abuse and neglect, Nayda found that a degree of ambiguity as to how this role was carried out in practice still existed. One of the key findings from the study was that participants did not always report their suspicions or cases where they knew child abuse and neglect were an issue. The author reported that the actions of nurses were motivated by what they considered to be the best outcomes for the children. Participants' actions were also influenced by a desire to protect the family from any negative outcomes or inappropriate responses of child protection services (Nayda 2002). At the same time they were also wary of imposing their own values on families, and feared the loss of the therapeutic relationship.

Participants' responses also pointed to a degree of hesitation in engaging in the process of consultation and confirmation with other agencies in cases of suspected abuse (Nayda 2002). This in part stemmed from the tension between nurses and other professionals as to who should report, indicating a general discomfort with this role. Participants reported that child protection workers' responses to their concerns were inconsistent, especially in situations of emotional abuse and neglect. In these situations participants reported feeling inadequate, as providing support did not prevent on-going abuse. This finding demonstrates the impact of the wider organisational environment on practice. At the same time the autonomy experienced by nurses working in a community setting can increase either confidence or the experience of uncertainty.

The author concluded that given the important role nurses have in relation to child protection, the concerns about intervening and reporting expressed by nurses needed to be addressed. The small sample size involved in the study undertaken by Nayda (2002) means that a degree of caution has to be exercised in relation to the claims that can be made of the findings. Nayda (2002) herself notes that it was not her intention that the findings should be viewed as representative of the experiences of all registered nurses in South Australia. Neither can it be assumed that the experiences reported in this study reflect those of nurses working in a different country. This does not negate the evidence as demonstrated by past and recent well-publicised cases of child abuse that have resulted in the death of a child.

RISK ASSESSMENT AND PROFESSIONAL PRACTICE

For nurses and midwives, the act of assessment has been pivotal in the role of care provision. Before any clinical intervention can be initiated, a thorough assessment of patient need is required. This same process is vital to supporting children and families under stress.

However, for some time, the act of assessing risk experienced by children and their families has often been viewed as something that takes place within the community setting. Identifying the potential for harm towards children is every nurse and midwife's responsibility. National guidance, across all four home nations, clearly identifies the actions required in the prevention or reduction of significant harm experienced by children.

Nurses and midwives in every setting see families under stress. While circumstances may not always provide an opportunity for a thorough assessment of an individual child's circumstances or how their family cope with any residual problems after illness, all nurses, regardless of setting, have a responsibility as members of healthcare staff. The Nursing and Midwifery Council in their code of conduct state that nurses and midwives have a duty 'to work with others to protect and promote the health and well-being of those in your care, their families and carers, and the wider community' (2008).

It is often during a period of crisis when families experience difficulties managing their children and other dependents. In such situations, a basic assessment of the conditions relating to the child, family or incident needs to be recorded. Information from other agencies should be gathered and multi-agency involvement commenced. Identifying and supporting children and families as early as possible have the potential to reduce the occurrence and impact of significant harm.

For a student or newly qualified nurse or midwife, identifying situations where potential or actual harm takes place can be daunting. However, guidance as to what needs to be done must be explicit and transparent. Effective supervision processes, record-keeping and continuous professional development and multi-professional working are common elements in clinical areas where child safeguarding practices underpin healthcare delivery. Every clinical area in primary and secondary care and the private sector have identified personnel with responsibility for advising on all aspects of child safeguarding and protection. Just as important as identifying the fire escapes within a new clinical area, so too is locating the lead clinician with responsibility for advising on child safeguarding matters.

While, as is often the case, practitioners in some clinical settings do not carry out a thorough assessment of risk, their observations and recordings contribute to the assessment process. The same processes of analysis and synthesis are required before decisions can be made as to what should happen next.

CASE STUDY

A 6-year-old boy, having been seen by the orthoptist, was travelling in the lift to the exit with an older female adult. A nurse sharing the lift witnessed the adult threatening and swearing at the boy. The adult pushed the boy hard across the lift after which the boy apparently looked quite frightened and was cowering in the corner of the lift.

The nurse did not intervene at this stage as she judged that challenging the adult in the confined space of the lift was inadvisable in relation to her own safety and the danger of exacerbating the situation. However, as soon as the lift was on the ground floor the nurse got in the next lift up, guessing that as the child had got into the lift on the 3rd floor and that he had most likely been attending the orthoptic clinic. She told the orthoptist in charge of the clinic what had happened and found out who the child was. They reported it to the nurse in charge of the children's ward, who accompanied them to the ground floor where they found the adult and child at the shop. They asked the adult if they could have a word with her. She agreed reluctantly and after a few minutes it was quite evident that the woman, who was the child's maternal grandmother, was not in good health and was struggling to cope with the four children left in her care while their single mother was serving a 12-month sentence in prison for drug offences.

Outcome

As a result of the nurse's action, social services were able to provide a package of care using voluntary agencies and members of the community to ensure that support was in place for the grandmother and the children. Through prison welfare services the mother was involved in the care plan and preparation was made for her release later that year.

The case study above is intended to demonstrate that protecting children is not 'rocket science' and is often down to observation, accountability and responsibility.

QUALITY ISSUES IN RISK ASSESSMENT AND MANAGEMENT PROCESSES

The assessment framework can be used by practitioners from all universal services, for example social services, healthcare, education and law enforcement. The framework is considered sufficiently broad to enable practitioners to share understanding through what has been termed a 'common language' (White et al. 2009). However, there is evidence highlighting that not all professionals have the same level of knowledge, understanding and confidence to fully assess all domains of the assessment framework (White et al. 2009). The findings from White et al.'s study, in tandem with the work of others (Gillingham and Humphreys 2010) suggest that not all practitioners with responsibility for child safeguarding and protection are prepared with the sufficient knowledge, skills and empathic understanding to undertake a rigorous risk assessment. It would be wrong to suggest that the assessment framework is the cause for this variation in practice. It is the quality of preparation and application of all practitioners that needs to be considered.

One of the issues impacting on the quality of the assessment process and the overall management of risk are the applied analytical skills of practitioners during and following the assessment. Analysis is an important cognitive activity where all factors or elements underpinning a root cause or causes are considered (Reber and Reber 2001). Analysis therefore is about making sense of the information gathered during the assessment and is followed by synthesis which involves considering all the factors or elements and combining them into an integrated whole (Reber and Reber 2001). Applying analysis and synthesis when assessing risk of significant harm therefore supports robust judgement and decision making as to whether there are unmet needs placing the child at significant risk of harm. If so, consideration has to be given to early interventions and multi-professional expertise.

Past procedural and management strategies have not encouraged practitioners in child care and protection to use their analytical skills. However, with contemporary child welfare policy there is an expectation that all practitioners with responsibilities for child safeguarding and protection need to develop and apply analytical thinking in decision making (Munro 2011). Helm (2009) identified a number of barriers influencing the application of analytical thinking in practice.

By applying an ecological framework to Helm's critique, from an individual perspective, some professionals would welcome greater preparation to maximise the use of analysis in practice. It is sometimes the subjective moral attributes of individuals within organisations which reduce objective assessment supported by analytical thinking (Hoyle 2008). There are also group barriers to the use of analysis. This is especially a concern with multi-professional working, when practitioners need to meet and discuss assessments, events and interventions. At an organisational level, a further barrier identified by Helm (2009) in the use of analysis is the part played by organisations that socialise and prepare practitioners to function. Education and practice is often guided by resources, organisational and managerial values, and social expectations. If practitioners are not using their analytical skills during risk assessments for whatever reason, they will not be in a position to synthesis the gathered data or to make appropriate and robust decisions.

These barriers raise a number of questions at different levels, highlighting areas which potentially threaten the quality of the wider assessment process. First, is the quality of preparation at undergraduate level sufficient to ensure that practitioners develop analytical thinking skills as well as the confidence to apply them in their daily practice? Second, are there sufficient opportunities for practitioners from all services to work together to develop their analytical skills? Third, at an organisational level, are organisational structures sufficient to support practitioners to address contemporary child welfare policies? Fourth, do organisations impress their own values and beliefs on practitioners, which may or may not support multi-professional working and analytical thinking? A final point regarding organisational involvement is the quality of supervision and leadership which is recognised as having an impact on practice (Helm 2009).

The need for a 'common language' must be addressed to ensure seamless practice, including the use and application of analysis across differing professional groups in order that the same level of application, transparency and robustness of risk management is evident. However, there are also further quality issues relating to the use of tools to support the assessment and decision making process.

While the framework provides a broad map of what to assess, further tools have been developed and used to explore specific processes of assessment. In a systematic review Barlow et al. (2012) appraised the tools used to support risk assessment as well those used to improve decision making. The authors identified a number of limitations. First, some tools were developed and put into practice without effectiveness being established. Second, not all tools were sufficiently aligned with the assessment framework. A final limitation noted by Barlow et al. was the lack of practitioner preparation to use and apply such tools in a safe, skilled and effective manner.

The conclusion of Barlow et al.'s systematic review identified the need for further research to ensure that tools developed to identify children's exposure to significant harm are reliable and valid for use in practice and that practitioners were prepared with the correct level of knowledge and skills to use such tools in a safe manner. Barlow et al. identified and reported a number of criteria for an ideal system of tools for assessment and decision making, presented below.

Criteria for an ideal system of tools for assessment and decision making

- Provide a balance of structure in terms of the use of professional judgement and standardised tools, in order to enable structured professional judgement to be employed:

  o to avoid erosion of professional competence and confidence;
  o to ensure that complexity is not minimised; and
  o to increase the accuracy of identifying whether a child is suffering, or is likely to suffer, significant harm and whether there is a likelihood of that harm recurring.

- Encourage assessment and analysis of information, which covers the full range of assessment domains that are known to be associated with children's optimal development, and thereby consistent with the assessment framework (Department of Health 2000).
- Be sensitive to the issue of different stages within an assessment:

  o either through the provision of a suite of tools to be used at different stages;
  o or the clear specification of at which stage and when the tools should be used during the process of an assessment (e.g. either at referral, assessment/section 47 enquiry or at the stage of return home or placement).

- Incorporate clear guidance with regard to assessing parental 'capacity to change' using both standardised assessment/diagnostic tools and goal-setting within agreed timeframes (Dawe and Harnett 2007).
- Provide guidance or pointers about how the model of structured professional judgement could be incorporated or integrated into a whole system in terms of:

  o organisational management;
  o implementation within a geographic area;
  o training and continuing professional development issues, including management of staff turnover; and
  o specific guidance as to how the model or tool is to be employed in the context of supervision.

Source: Barlow et al. (2012: 11).

While this systematic review focused on the English perspective, other nations using similar tools to identify children exposed to significant harm need to be aware of the limitations imposed by using such instruments.

To support practitioners responsible for assessing risk in children's lives, Broadhurst et al. have updated an original document produced before the introduction of assessment frameworks now used across all home nations. The document entitled *Ten*

Pitfalls and How to Avoid Them: What Research Tells Us (2010) was part of *Assessing Risk in Child Protection*, an NSPCC Policy Practice Research Series report first published in 1998 (Cleaver et al. 1998). The second edition, like the first, is informed by research and guides practitioners on how best to avoid common errors that in the past have contributed to poor decision making. Broadhurst et al. raise once more the need for practitioners to use 'critical thinking' and 'reflexive awareness' in an effort to avoid the 'error-trap' in practice. Guidance is presented for both practitioner and manager. The authors' state that:

> Risk must be managed on each and every occasion through careful consideration of both case-specific and research evidence. This revised booklet offers practitioners an accessible guide to research evidence to support the second half of this equation. Research-informed practice provides a useful counter balance to intuitive or gut reasoning. The guidance will be very useful for newly qualified practitioners, but will also serve as an aide-mémoire for the more experienced. (2010: 5)

A brief summary of Broadhurst et al.'s ten pitfalls is given below.

Ten pitfalls and how to avoid them: What research tells us (Broadhurst et al. 2010)

1. An initial hypothesis is formulated on the basis of incomplete information, and is assessed and accepted too quickly. Practitioners become committed to this hypothesis and do not seek out information that may disconfirm or refute it.

2. Information taken at the first enquiry is not adequately recorded, facts are not checked and there is a failure to feedback the outcome to the referrer.

3. Attention is focused on the most visible or pressing problems; case history and less 'obvious' details are insufficiently explored.

4. Insufficient weight is given to information from family, friends and neighbours.

5. Insufficient attention is paid to what children say, how they look and how they behave.

6. There is insufficient full engagement with parents (mothers/fathers/other family carers) to assess risk.

7. Initial decisions that are overly focused on age categories of children can result in older children being left in situations of unacceptable risk.

8. There is insufficient support/supervision to enable practitioners to work effectively with service users who are unco-operative, ambivalent, confrontational, avoidant or aggressive.

9. Throughout the initial assessment process, professionals do not clearly check that others have understood their communication. There is an assumption that information shared is information understood.

10. Case responsibility is diluted in the context of multi-agency working, impacting both on referrals and response. The local authority may inappropriately signpost families to other agencies, with no follow up.

The full document can be accessed by visiting www.nspcc.org.uk/research.

EMERGING THEMES

Risk assessment contributes to the wider activity of managing risk, including decision making. The outcome of this process may lead to the introduction of early interventions as well as the inclusion of specific services supported by other professionals. Education to prepare nurses and midwives to contribute to the assessment process is necessary to ensure that they have an understanding of the main theories underpinning the assessment framework, as well as knowledge of the factors that impact on the quality of the assessment outcome.

Practitioners in healthcare require skills in critical analysis and synthesis when assessing the needs of children and their families. The level of analysis and synthesis will impact on the quality of assessing risk and the wider management of risk. Leaders and managers overseeing the practice of nurses and midwives are responsible for ensuring that all practitioners in their team are prepared, supervised and resourced to facilitate quality risk management in their day-to-day practice. A further theme is the need to prepare practitioners to work jointly with other professionals to meet the needs of children and their families. In order to reduce role ambiguity and to increase the effectiveness of multi-professional working, joint education and development is required at both undergraduate and post-qualifying levels.

Possibly a final theme identified in this chapter is the need for further robust research into the use of specific tools to aid aspects of the assessment process.

CONCLUSION

This chapter has addressed a number of elements that impact on risk assessment and the wider concept of risk management. Child maltreatment is a preventable occurrence requiring a contemporary public health approach and associated strategies to manage prevention, as well as universal and targeted interventions. Assessing risk for any child is the first step in that process. Practitioners are not always prepared to fulfil their roles or responsibilities, just as other multi-professionals can be equally hesitant.

The risk management process has been presented, which highlighted the activities of analysis and synthesis. Factors that impact on the quality of the risk assessment process have also been discussed. Evidence on how to avoid making errors during the process of assessing risk has brought the chapter to a close.

FURTHER READING AND INFORMATION

Barlow, J., Fisher, J. and Jones, D. (2012) *Systematic Review of Models of Analysing Significant Harm: Research Report DFE-RR199*. London: Department for Education. Available at: www.gov.uk/government/uploads/system/uploads/attachment_data/file/183949/DFE-RR199.pdf (accessed 20 December 2013).

Bostock, L., Bairstow, S., Fish, S. and MacLeod, F. (2005) *Managing Risk and Minimising Mistakes in Services to Children and Families: Children and Families' Services Report 6*. Bristol: Social Care Institute for Excellence. Available at: www.scie.org.uk/publications/reports/report06.pdf (accessed 20 December 2013).

Broadhurst, K., White, S., Fish, S., Munro, E., Fletcher, K. and Lincoln, H. (2010) *Ten Pitfalls and How to Avoid Them: What Research Tells Us*. London: NSPCC. Available at: www.nspcc.org.uk/inform/research/findings/tenpitfalls_wda78613.html (accessed 20 December 2013).

Scottish Government (2012) *National Framework to Support the Assessment of Children and Young People*. Edinburgh: Crown. Available at: www.scotland.gov.uk/Publications/2012/11/7143 (accessed 20 December 2013).

REFERENCES

Barlow, J., Fisher, J., Jones, D. (2012) *Systematic Review of Models of Analysing Significant Harm*. London: Department for Education. p. 31.

Belsky, J. (1993) Etiology of maltreatment: a developmental-ecological analysis. *Psychological Bulletin* 114(3): 413–434.

Broadhurst, K., White, S., Fish, S., Munro, E., Fletcher, K. and Lincoln, H. (2010) *Ten Pitfalls and How to Avoid Them: What Research Tells Us*. London: NSPCC. Available at: www.nspcc.org.uk/inform/research/findings/tenpitfalls_wda78613.html (accessed 20 December 2013).

Bronfenbrenner, U. (1979) *The Ecology of Human Development: Experiments by Nature and Design*. London: Harvard University Press.

Cleaver, H., Wattam, C., Cawson, P., and Gordon, R. (1998) Ten pitfalls and how to avoid them: what research tells us. *Assessing Risk in Child Protection*. London: NSPCC Policy Practice Research Series Report.

Crisp, B. and Lister, P. (2004) Child protection and public health nurse's responsibilities. *Journal of Advanced Nursing* 476: 656–665.

Dawe, S. and Harnett, P. H. (2007) Improving family functioning in methadone maintained families: Results from a randomised controlled trial. *Journal of Substance Abuse Treatment* 32: 381–90.

Department of Health (2000) Framework for the Assessment of Children in Need and their Families. London: The Stationery Office. Available at: http://webarchive.nationalarchives.gov.uk/+/www.dh.gov.uk/en/publicationsandstatistics/publications/publicationspolicy-andguidance/dh_4003256 (accessed January 2012).

Gilbert, R., Fluke, J., O'Donnell, M., Gonzalez-Izquierdo, A., Brownell, M., Gulliver, P., Janson, S. and Sidebotham, P. (2012) Child maltreatment: variation in trends and policies in six developed countries. *Lancet* 379: 758–772.

Gillingham, P. and Humphreys, C. (2010) Child protection practitioners and decision-making tools: observations and reflections from the front line. *British Journal of Social Work* 40: 2598–2616.

Grey, M. and Sarangi, J. (2003) Protecting the public's health. In J. Orme., P. Taylor, T. Harrison, M. Grey (eds), *Public Health for the 21st Century*. Maidenhead: Open University Press pp. 107–127.

Helm, D. (2009) *Analysis and Getting it Right for Every Child: A Discussion Paper*. Stirling: University of Stirling.

Horwath, J. (2010) *The Child's World: The Comprehensive Guide to Assessing Children in Need*. London: Jessica Kingsley.

Hoyle, D. (2008) *Problematizing Every Child Matters*. Infed. Available at: www.infed.org/socialwork/every_child_matters_a_critique.htm (accessed January 2012).

Laming, Lord (2003) *The Victoria Climbié Inquiry*. London: HMSO.

Masten, A. and Gewirtz, A. (2009) *Vulnerability and Resilience in Early Child Development*, In K. McCartney and D. Phillips (ed.), *Blackwell Handbook of Early Childhood Development*. Oxford: Blackwell.

Munro, E. (2011) *The Munro Review of Child Protection: Final Report: A child-centred system*. London: Department for Education.

Nayda R. (2002) Influences on registered nurses' decision-making in cases of suspected child abuse. *Child Abuse Review* 11: 168–178.

Nursing and Midwifery Council (2008) *The Code: Standards of Conduct, Performance and Ethics for Nurses and Midwives*. London: Nursing and Midwifery Council.

O'Donnell, M. and Scott, D. (2008) Child abuse and neglect – is it time for a public health approach? *Austrilia and New Zealand Public Health Journal* 32: 325–330.

Reber, A. and Reber, E. (2001) *The Penguin Dictionary of Psychology*. London: Penguin.

Scottish Executive (2000) *Protecting Children: A Shared Responsibility*. Edinburgh: Crown.

Sidebotham, P. and Weeks, M. (2010) Multidisciplinary contributions to assessment of children in need. In J. Horwath (ed.), *The Child's World: The Comprehensive Guide to Assessing Children in Need*. London: Jessica Kingsley.

White, S., Hall, C. and Peckover, S. (2009) The descriptive tyranny of the common assessment framework: technologies of categorization and professional practice in child welfare. *British Journal of Social Work* 39: 1197–1217.

PART 2

RELATIONSHIPS, COMMUNICATION AND PRACTICE

5

VULNERABILITY IN PREGNANCY AND CHILDBIRTH

JOAN CAMERON

CHAPTER SUMMARY

While risk has been a central feature of the organisation and management of care in pregnancy and childbirth for decades, the concept of social vulnerability is emerging as an important feature in enhancing the outcomes of care for women, their babies and families. The importance of understanding how individual women perceive and deal with risks and stresses in their lives is central to care provision. An asset-based approach to care appreciates the perspective of the woman. It facilitates a partnership approach, which means that care is personalised and flexible.

Women who experience social exclusion are at increased risk of mortality (Lewis 2007). The same is true of their unborn babies (Lewis 2007). Barriers to care for women who are vulnerable include language difficulties and cultural stereotyping (Reynolds and Shams 2005; Straus et al. 2009), feeling awkward (Hall and van Teijlingen 2006); lack of knowledge or understanding on the part of the caregiver (Tsianakas and Liamputtong 2002; Raeside 2003; Mezey et al. 2003). There is a growing body of evidence that care individualised to meet the needs of the woman can enhance the outcome for both mother and baby (Leggate 2008; National Collaborating Centre for Women's and Children's Health 2010).

Health professionals working with pregnant women must seek to understand the context of their lives. An asset-based approach to care recognises and builds on strengths and facilitates partnership working. It can allow poverty, social exclusion and lifestyle factors to be addressed with the aim of enhancing outcomes for women, babies and their families (Maternity Services Action Group 2011).

This chapter will explore how vulnerability in pregnancy and childbirth relates to vulnerability in infancy. Importantly, it will consider how health and social care professionals can work with women and families to enhance outcomes of care in partnership.

AIMS OF THIS CHAPTER

This chapter will enable understanding of the relationship between vulnerability during and after pregnancy and childbirth and child protection.

Learning outcomes

After reading this chapter and following a period of reflection the reader will be able to:

- Identify women and families who are vulnerable during and after pregnancy and childbirth.
- Compare and contrast risk-based and vulnerability based approaches to child protection.
- Evaluate and apply an asset-based approach to child protection, within the context of pregnancy and childbirth.
- Recognise the challenges and benefits of inter-professional working.

Key words

asset-based approach; pregnancy; risk; social vulnerability

Pregnancy and childbirth are important life events for women, babies and families. The dominant theme in pregnancy and child protection relates to risk (Stahl and Hundley 2003; Bryers and van Teijlingen 2010). The concept of risk in the context of pregnancy and child protection refers to the potential for harm. This includes: determining if the woman or child is 'at risk', estimating the level of risk and providing care based on the perception of risk. The risk-based approach to care has been challenged as focusing only on narrow parameters and failing to take into account the wider social and cultural aspects that impact on the lives of women and families

(Downe 2010). This, it has been suggested, leads to inappropriate intervention which fails to meet the needs of women and their families (Downe 2010).

An emerging approach within pregnancy and childbirth is the concept of social vulnerability. Social vulnerability has been defined as:

> The exposure to contingencies and stress, and difficulty in coping with them. Vulnerability thus has two sides: an external side of risks, shocks and stress to which an individual or household is subject; and an internal side which is defencelessness, meaning a lack of means to cope without damaging loss. (Chambers 1989: 2)

Sabates-Wheeler and Haddad (2005) suggest that both the exposure to risks and stress and the ability to cope with risks and stress need to be considered, as it is the imbalance between the two that increases social vulnerability. While tools are being developed to measure vulnerability, it must be acknowledged that vulnerability is not static but constantly changing (World Bank 2012). Furthermore, vulnerability is not an objective measurement. How an individual perceives a situation affects their responses to it. This means that responses to social vulnerability must be personalised and flexible.

Reflective activity

Based on your experience, consider what factors might be associated with vulnerability in pregnancy.

Women may become pregnant because they are vulnerable or they may be vulnerable because they are pregnant (Newman and Newman 2009). Women who are vulnerable may include those who have experienced sexual abuse or domestic abuse, as well as those living in poverty or social exclusion or who have lifestyle behaviours such as illicit drug use which can impact adversely on their health and well-being and that of their children (Cuthbert et al. 2011). An asset-based approach or needs-based approach to care seeks to understand the perspective of the woman and to work in partnership with her and her family. This approach recognises and builds on strengths. Importantly, the role of poverty, social exclusion and lifestyle behaviours including drug use can be addressed within these approaches and may help improve outcomes for women, their babies and families (Leggate 2008).

CONTEXTUALISING THE CHALLENGE

Pregnancy and childbirth are usually times of great joy in a family. In the United Kingdom, the majority of women are healthy and give birth to healthy babies. However, in a small number of cases, pregnancy and childbirth may present overwhelming challenges to women and their families, and the health and well-being of the baby may be jeopardised. Pregnancy, childbirth and the postnatal period are times of transition and, as such, can present challenges to women and their families (Deave et al. 2008). The majority of women and families make the transition successfully, albeit with support from health professionals, family and community support (Ward and Mitchell 2004). Some parents, however, experience significant challenges during pregnancy and afterwards. Circumstances which appear to have an adverse effect on the transition process include very young mothers (Cater and Coleman 2006), parents who misuse substances (Dunn et al. 2002; Gorin 2004), domestic abuse (Wiemann et al. 2000; Cloutier et al. 2002), parents or children with learning disabilities (Morris 2003) and parents experiencing mental health problems (Royal College of Psychiatrists 2011). In these circumstances, midwives and other professionals working with pregnant and newly delivered women may find themselves working to promote and ensure the well-being of the baby and family (CEMACH 2011).

Increasingly midwives are the first point of contact for women accessing the maternity services. They often form strong relationships with women and their families, and their intimate views of family life can help them to identify situations where the rights of the child may be threatened. However, the link between the woman and the midwife may also present challenges with regard to upholding the rights of the baby. Midwives may experience role conflict as they try to combine support for the woman with surveillance. The dissonance experienced by health professionals undertaking child protection and support is widely reported and can be an influential factor in failing to acknowledge babies and children at risk of harm (Chapman 2002; Ellefsen 2002; Keys 2005; Piltz and Wachtel 2009).

RISK OR VULNERABILITY

The traditional approach to maternity care in the United Kingdom is based around the concept of risk, where a woman is allocated a risk category based on certain medical or social characteristics. The perception of pregnancy as normal only in retrospect has been subject to extensive critique (van Teijlingen 2005). In particular, it is associated with high rates of interventions which may actually increase the risk of harm to the woman or the baby (Johanson et al. 2002). Women have also complained that the risk-based approach is depersonalising and fails to take account of individual circumstances which may lessen the risks (Redshaw and Heikkila 2010). The risk-based approach has also been adopted for child protection where babies or children are identified as being 'at risk' of harm. This approach has been associated with a dependence on procedures and protocols which may reduce contact between professionals and children, increase intrusive child protection procedures and fail babies and children in need because they are perceived as not being at risk of serious abuse (Lord Laming 2009; Munro 2011).

> **Reflective activity**
>
> From your experience, what are the challenges of using an estimate of risk to determine care in pregnancy and childbirth?

Problems with any risk-based approach include the potential for false positives and false negatives. This is equally true of a risk-based approach in child protection. False positive outcomes can result in inappropriate intervention and may cause harm to the baby and family. False negative outcomes are associated with harm to the baby as families who would benefit from support are not recognised. Sibert et al. (2007) critiqued the evidence base for child protection after a leading article in the *British Medical Journal* by an American paediatrician described it as 'well established' and 'robust' (Chadwick 2006). They found that the assertions were based on an extensive list of citations that failed to stand up to critical scrutiny. The lack of a robust evidence base further complicates the situation for health professionals when trying to predict or identify risky situations.

The concept of vulnerability relates to the individual and their environment (Sabates-Wheeler and Haddad 2005). It recognises that for some women, being pregnant or having other social or environmental challenges means that they are less able to care for their child. It does not always mean that they are unable to make judgements or provide care but that they would benefit from support, and this could reduce the potential for harm to the baby. Asset-based or needs-based approaches to care focus on identifying the resources that an individual or family possess that promote health and well-being. This enables health and social care practitioners to work with the woman and her family to enhance health outcomes. These approaches currently inform much of the child protection work throughout the United Kingdom (Cuthbert et al. 2011).

RECOGNISING VULNERABILITY

A range of circumstances are associated with vulnerability in pregnancy. Changing family structures where one 'parent' is not biologically related to the child are associated with an increase in the probability of child abuse occurring. Other factors include being the first or youngest child. Certain characteristics of the child also increase their vulnerability and the possibility of child abuse occurring. These include illness or disability. Recognition of vulnerability enables specific interventions to enhance self-esteem and promote health and well-being. A potential benefit of an asset-based approach to protecting babies is that it enables women and families to identify the knowledge, skills, support and potential they have, rather than simply considering what they lack. An asset-based approach allows midwives to work with women and families to develop individualised, person-centred responses to situations. This approach may help reduce the dissonance and conflict experienced by midwives involved in circumstances where they have formed a relationship with the woman and her family and where they recognise that the environment is potentially harmful to the new-born infant.

POVERTY AND SOCIAL DEPRIVATION

Poverty and social deprivation are associated with a range of issues that impact on pregnancy and increase the potential for harm to the child (Dennison 2004; Collingwood Bakeo and Clarke 2006). These include low birth weight, which is defined as a birth weight of less than 2500 grams. Low birth weight may be due to shortened duration of pregnancy or poor intrauterine growth. Both are associated with physical and cognitive disability (Collingwood Bakeo and Clarke 2006; Griggs and Walker 2008). Morbidity associated with low birth weight includes cerebral palsy and developmental delay, chronic lung disease, sight and hearing impairment. An association has been demonstrated between the morbidity caused by low birth-weight and increased financial stress and decreased mental health and well-being of parents (Mak and Ho 2007; Hassall et al. 2005; Baker et al. 2003). Having a child with a disability may also be associated with stigmatisation and discrimination (Carnevale 2007).

CASE STUDY

Sam was born at 25 weeks gestation after his mother went into labour prematurely. He was in the neonatal intensive care unit for almost eight months. As a result of his prematurity, he has chronic lung disease. When he was discharged home from the neonatal intensive care unit, he needed additional oxygen delivered via nasal cannula. If the family want to go out with Sam, they have to carry an oxygen cylinder in the pram. The worry of running out of oxygen when they are out means that Sam's mother usually stays at home. Sam is difficult to feed because of his lung problems and he needs to have some of his feeds given by nasogastric tube. Because of Sam's breathing and feeding difficulties he is a poor sleeper, waking every 2–3 hours. His parents have been counselled by medical staff about the possibility of long-term problems such as problems with visual and hearing loss, as well as the risk of cerebral palsy. The full extent of the morbidity associated with Sam's preterm birth may not be known until he is much older, so his parents have to cope with an uncertain future for Sam and for themselves.

RESPONSE: SUPPORTING SAM AND HIS FAMILY

Sam's family are vulnerable because he has additional care needs. Babies with chronic lung disease are prone to frequent respiratory infections which may require hospital treatment (Greenough et al. 2001). Sam's parents may have to alter their work patterns to care for him. One parent may have to stay at home, rather than work outside the home. His parents may also still be trying to deal with the financial costs associated with having a baby in a neonatal intensive care unit (Hodek et al. 2011).

While Sam is in the neonatal intensive care unit a number of interventions can help his parents form strong attachments with him. Teaching Sam's parents how to care for him and how to interpret his cues and interact with him can reduce parental stress. There is evidence to suggest that this approach promotes parents' self-reliance before babies are discharged home (Wielenga et al. 2000; Prentice and Stainton 2003). 'Kangaroo' care or skin-to-skin contact has been shown to reduce maternal anxiety significantly and increases feelings of competence in caring for the baby (Feldman et al. 2003). It has also been shown to increase mother–infant interaction and reduce postnatal depression (Feldman et al. 2003). Postnatal depression has been shown to impact on mother–infant attachment behaviours (see Chapter 3) and on infant development (Poobalan et al. 2007). Therefore interventions to reduce, recognise and treat postnatal depression may be important for both the woman and her baby.

Providing counselling and psychological interventions to promote relaxation while Sam is in the neonatal intensive care unit have also been shown to reduce the trauma felt by parents of preterm babies (Jotzo and Poets 2005). Even apparently meaningless or trivial 'chat' between parents and health professionals caring for preterm babies has been shown to increase mothers' confidence and their feeling of self-control in a very stressful environment (Fenwick et al. 2001).

Discharge preparation programmes that take a problem-solving approach have been shown to improve the way in which parents interact with their infant (Ortenstrand et al. 2001). Inviting the health visitor to visit the neonatal intensive care unit prior to the baby's discharge home and involving the multi-disciplinary team in discharge planning meetings have been associated with increased parental confidence in caring for their baby and enhanced feelings of support once the baby has been discharged home.

Home visiting by a community neonatal home care team may assist Sam's parents in developing confidence in dealing with respiratory infections in the home, thus reducing the need for Sam to be readmitted to hospital. The use of an apnoea monitor for Sam could decrease parental stress. This intervention has been shown to decrease stress in parents whose baby is at risk of apnoea (Brett et al. 2011). Health visitor support is important for the family. The health visitor will be able to monitor Sam's development and facilitate early intervention where developmental delay is noted. The provision of multi-disciplinary liaison with all those involved in Sam's care has been shown to reduce stress and enhance coping skills for mothers (Brett et al. 2011).

The third sector is another potential source of support for Sam's family. Several organisations provide support for preterm babies and their families and can be a valuable source of peer support. The charity Bliss provides information, peer support and counselling for parents of preterm babies. They have a network of support groups which Sam's parents may be able to attend or link with. As Sam's diagnosis evolves, organisations such as Contact A Family may also be useful to them. The evidence base shows that parents of preterm infants value support from 'experienced' parents. Parents with experience of caring for preterm babies are sources of information and emotional support for new parents. They also act as role models, and new parents can draw 'strength' from their example (Brett et al. 2011).

Caring for a baby with complex needs at home can be stressful for parents. Low birth weight is recognised as a significant factor in child abuse and neglect (Sidebotham et al. 2006). However, implementing supportive interventions commenced while a baby is in the neonatal intensive care unit and continuing to provide access to information and support from a range of sources can enhance developmental outcomes for the baby and increase parental interaction and satisfaction with their role.

TEENAGE PREGNANCY AND PARENTING

Teenage pregnancy has a strong association with poverty and social deprivation (Harden et al. 2009). Antecedents of teenage pregnancy include lack of support at home or in school, family conflict and breakdown, violence in the home and sexual abuse (Harden et al. 2009). Significant numbers of teenagers who become parents are likely to have been in care or fostered (Haydon 2003). Teenage pregnancy and parenting is associated with low self-esteem and low educational achievement (Wellings 2001).

Teenage fathers are more likely to report being exposed to violent punishment and sexual abuse during childhood. They are also more likely to report mental health problems and to drink, smoke and misuse substances (Department of Health 2008). Young fathers are also reported to be more likely to be involved with the criminal justice system (Thornberry et al. 2009).

Teenagers who become pregnant are more likely to smoke (Hamlyn et al. 2002), have poor nutrition and are more likely to live in poverty (Department of Health 2008). They are more likely to give birth to a low birth weight baby (Jolly et al. 2000). Babies born to teenage mothers have a higher mortality rate than babies born to older mothers (Botting et al. 1998). Evidence suggests that babies born to teenage parents are more likely to experience maltreatment and neglect than babies born to older parents (Afifi and Brownridge 2008; Lounds et al. 2006). Long-term outcomes for children born to teenage parents suggest that they are more likely to have emotional and behavioural problems and have an increased risk of being harmed. Ultimately, they are more likely to become teenage parents (Corlyon and Stock 2011).

CASE STUDY

Selma is 13. She has an appointment with the midwife to book pregnancy care. She arrives at the antenatal clinic with her mother. She thinks she is about 12 weeks pregnant. She lives with her mother and stepfather and her two younger brothers. Her stepfather is unaware that she is pregnant.

RESPONSE: SUPPORTING SELMA

As well as considering Selma's need for antenatal care, the midwife has to consider other issues such as safeguarding when undertaking the booking interview. Selma is below the age of consent so the midwife will want to explore the circumstances in which Selma became pregnant, and the age of her partner. Maternity services will usually invoke a safeguarding pathway for very young teenagers and many will have a specialist antenatal care assessment protocol and pathway which will assess the health and social needs of teenagers who become pregnant and provide appropriate services to support them. For example, specialist education services may be available during and after pregnancy.

Tailored antenatal and postnatal support may be available. Teenagers who become pregnant are more likely to smoke. This has long-term implications for their health but can also affect the development of the baby in utero. Most maternity services provide smoking cessation support. However, for Selma, who is living at home, a family-centred approach may be appropriate.

Because Selma is very young, she is at greater risk of giving birth to a low birth weight baby. Tailored antenatal care that provides continuity and which she perceives as meeting her needs means that Selma is more likely to attend care appointments, which in turn allows for timely intervention. Young women who are pregnant often report that attitudes of health professionals deter them from attending and seeking professional help. It is essential that all members of the multi-disciplinary team understand the importance of an inclusive approach in enhancing outcomes for teenage parents and their babies.

Housing is important for all parents. Teenage parents, however, are more likely to have housing problems which can, in turn, affect their emotional well-being and their relationship with their baby. Selma's situation needs to be assessed with regard to housing needs after the baby is born. Social Services may be required to provide assistance with accommodation and support, especially if Selma's parents are unable or unwilling to have her and the baby in their home.

Tailored services to promote effective parenting skills for teenage parents include Sure Start, Family Nurse Partnership and third sector initiatives. There is a growing body of evidence demonstrating that these are effective in enabling teenage parents to develop interactive skills to promote attachment with the baby (Department of Health 2008). These interventions have also been shown to be helpful in reducing postnatal depression and feelings of isolation experienced by teenage parents.

Much of the care will be focused on Selma and her baby. Teenage fathers have reported feeling excluded from pregnancy care, which influences their experience of fatherhood and their ability to parent successfully (Quinton et al. 2002; Bunting and McAuley 2004). This is regrettable as there is a growing body of evidence demonstrating that young fathers want to be involved with their baby and find that the experience of being a father gives their life meaning (Quinton et al. 2002; McDonnell et al. 2009). There is also evidence that being involved with their baby reduces their involvement in delinquent behaviour in the long-term, with young men citing their responsibility for their baby as being a 'wake-up' call (Thornberry et al. 2009).

Teenage mothers can also benefit from the involvement of the baby's father in the postnatal period. There is evidence that they experience better mental health and well-being when the father is supportive and involved in the baby's care (Gee and Rhodes 2003). Supported teenage mothers are also more likely to demonstrate positive child attachment behaviours and childrearing skills, which, in turn, lead to enhanced mothering and a decrease in behavioural difficulties in children (Berrington et al. 2005).

There is a paucity of good-quality evidence from the United Kingdom relating to strategies to support teenage fathers. Evidence from the United States suggests that community based interventions using a needs-based approach with one-to-one coaching is effective in developing fathering skills (Bronte-Tinkew et al. 2008). These need to be piloted and evaluated in the United Kingdom to test their appropriateness with different groups and in a range of social and environmental contexts.

Teenage parents are vulnerable because of their age, as well as experiencing many social and environmental obstacles. These can impact adversely on the well-being and development of their baby. However, they also have the potential to develop supportive relationships to nurture their infant and to encourage them to grow and develop. Inclusive, community based approaches that are tailored to the individual needs of teenage parents are more likely to achieve positive outcomes and enhance the well-being of the parents and their baby.

GENDER-BASED VIOLENCE

Gender-based violence is a term that encompasses a wide range of abuse which is experienced disproportionately by women and perpetrated predominantly by men. Domestic abuse is part of the spectrum of gender-based violence. Domestic abuse includes physical violence as well as emotional and psychological abuse. Although it can occur in any setting, there are strong associations between domestic abuse and poverty, homelessness and mental health problems. There is evidence that pregnancy can be a trigger for domestic abuse and that it is associated with symptoms of depression in women in the antenatal and postnatal period, as well as violence in the postnatal period (Flach et al. 2011).

Domestic abuse can harm the fetus. It has been shown to cause miscarriage, premature birth, fetal injury and stillbirth. It is also associated with behavioural problems in a child at 18 months of age (Flach et al. 2011). Brandon et al. (2008) found that there was a relationship between domestic violence and child abuse – in some cases leading to the death of the child.

There is evidence that pregnant women find being asked about domestic abuse as part of antenatal booking acceptable (Davidson et al. 2000; Price 2004). It is recommended that women should be offered the opportunity to disclose domestic abuse during pregnancy (Davidson et al. 2000). However, there is also evidence that midwives may be reluctant to question the woman about domestic abuse. Reasons for not asking women about domestic abuse include not wishing to cause offence, not knowing what to do, and identifying with a woman who discloses abuse.

Claudia is 30 years old. This is her third pregnancy and she is now 28 weeks pregnant. She is married and has one child who is four years old. Her last pregnancy ended in miscarriage. In her local maternity unit, midwives routinely ask about domestic abuse at the booking clinic. Information about domestic abuse is given to all women.

At booking Claudia said that she was not experiencing abuse at home. However, as the midwife carries out the antenatal check, she notices that Claudia has old bruises on her arms and a fresh bruise on her abdomen.

CASE STUDY

RESPONSE: SUPPORTING CLAUDIA

Claudia's midwife would benefit from having undertaken additional training in the identification and care of women who report domestic abuse (Salmon et al. 2006). This would enable her to ask Claudia if she was encountering situations where she was harmed or afraid at home. Even if Claudia chooses not to disclose on this occasion, the midwife should put the question to her again at key times during the pregnancy, including admission in labour. Having posters and information cards in different formats in the antenatal clinic advertising support for women experiencing domestic abuse will make Claudia aware of the range of services available to her. The midwife should also be alert to other possible indicators of domestic abuse such as missed appointments, the refusal of the partner to leave, and frequent visits to the GP or midwife with vague symptoms.

The design and implementation of a protocol and care pathway for women self-disclosing domestic abuse has been shown to be effective in increasing the number of women who disclose domestic abuse and who access support (Bacchus et al. 2010). Continuity of care would enhance Claudia's trust in the midwife and may help her disclose information that could be of use to her should she seek to take action to deal with the abuse. It is important that the midwife documents any disclosures Claudia makes in a way that is sensitive and protects her confidentiality (Bacchus et al. 2010). However, Claudia does need to understand that if she discloses information that suggests her child is at risk of abuse, the information will be shared with other agencies to safeguard the child.

Even if Claudia chooses not to take action, there is evidence that support from the midwife can enhance her sense of well-being. The midwife can offer information about support groups and encourage Claudia to have an 'escape plan' should the situation deteriorate. Taking a non-judgemental approach is important and this may be difficult for the midwife if she believes that Claudia should leave the relationship but chooses to stay.

There is an association between the severity of violence and the risk of violence to children living in the home. If the midwife is concerned about the safety and well-being of Claudia's existing child, then she is required to take action to ensure the child's safety. The local maternity unit may have a Supervisor of Midwives who can support the midwife in taking this action or they may have a named midwife with responsibility for child protection. The midwife should explain that the child may not be safe due to the levels of violence in the home.

Where child protection procedures are activated, Claudia may be at increased risk of abuse because of her disclosure. Multi-agency involvement at this time is essential to ensure that she is safe and supported. Documentation of any information Claudia gives, together with photographs of injuries, can be important in any court action. Domestic abuse is a criminal act and the perpetrator may be prosecuted, even if Claudia chooses not to give evidence. In these circumstances the notes that the midwife makes may be helpful in protecting Claudia and her child.

Evidence to support the use of interventions to reduce the incidence of domestic abuse is scarce. Sullivan and Bybee (1999) found that women who spent at least one night in a shelter followed by advocacy and counselling reported feeling safer and also experienced less abuse in the two-year period following the intervention. In the United States the use of permanent protective orders are associated with a decrease in the reported incidence of physical violence (Holt et al. 2002). However, the use of temporary protective orders is associated with a significant increase in psychological abuse, while the level of physical abuse is unchanged.

Domestic abuse is a significant event in pregnancy and is associated with harm to the woman, the fetus and dependent children. Routine enquiry and support by the midwife is helpful to the woman; however, where dependent children are at risk of harm, a multi-agency approach is essential. While the midwife's primary duty of care is to the woman, child protection legislation means that confidentiality may be breached by the midwife so that information to safeguard children is shared with relevant agencies.

LIFESTYLE BEHAVIOURS INCLUDING SUBSTANCE MISUSE

Some lifestyle behaviours can jeopardise the health and well-being of the woman and her family. Substance misuse is a serious and complex mental health disorder involving drugs or alcohol. It is associated with poor health outcomes for the woman and can impact on the development of the baby in utero and afterwards, because of its effect on parenting abilities (Cuthbert et al. 2011). Drug use is strongly associated with poverty and deprivation. Drug use is an important cause of maternal mortality in the United Kingdom. It places the woman at risk of contracting hepatitis B, hepatitis C and HIV. All of these can be transmitted to the fetus via the placenta. Drug use in pregnancy can result in miscarriage, preterm birth, growth retardation and congenital malformations in the fetus. Drug use is also associated with neonatal abstinence syndrome in the newborn infant. This is a collection of symptoms which affects babies born to mothers who are dependent on opiates, barbiturates and benzodiazepines. The baby may be irritable or hyperactive and have difficulty breathing and feeding.

As well as the physical complications of substance misuse, there may be social and environmental problems which can place the woman and her baby in danger. Procuring drugs can place the woman at risk of violence or sexually transmitted diseases. Women who substance misuse are also more likely to be in contact with the criminal justice system. There is little information on the fathers of these babies, although evidence suggests that more fathers substance misuse than mothers.

Alcohol use in pregnancy is associated with older women and those from managerial and professional backgrounds (Cuthbert et al. 2011). The level of alcohol consumed in pregnancy is generally low. However, a small number of women who become pregnant are dependent on alcohol and this makes them and their babies vulnerable to abuse.

Alcohol dependency in pregnancy can cause fetal alcohol syndrome, which is associated with low birth weight, learning difficulties and neurological abnormalities. Maternal alcohol dependency is also associated with neglect and long-term mental health problems in children. Parental alcohol misuse is strongly associated with infant death and injury during co-sleeping.

Asha is a 23-year-old woman who is pregnant for the second time. She has a history of substance misuse – she admits to injecting heroin as well binge drinking alcohol. Her first child was born four years ago and has been adopted. Her partner is in prison, awaiting trial on charges of drug dealing. Asha is currently living in hostel accommodation. She has expressed a wish to keep this baby and is anxious that the baby will be placed for adoption again. She also wants to come off heroin. Her parents have agreed to help her if she stops using drugs.

CASE STUDY

RESPONSE: SUPPORTING ASHA

Asha would benefit from support from a specialist midwife and the multi-disciplinary team, including obstetricians, social workers and addiction services. It is important that she avoids injecting heroin, so she will be encouraged to go onto a methadone treatment programme. Withdrawal from drugs is dangerous during pregnancy as it can cause severe fetal distress and even fetal death. Methadone is available legally and is free, so this will allow Asha to use any income to support herself rather than buying drugs.

Asha's alcohol intake will be assessed and she will be supported to address it through involvement with addiction services. Sudden cessation of alcohol intake in women who are heavy drinkers is associated with fetal distress and fetal loss. Asha will be offered screening for hepatitis B, C and HIV. This will allow appropriate support and treatment programmes to be commenced should she test positive for any of these. She will also be offered regular ultrasound scans to check the growth of the fetus, as drug misuse is associated with low birth weight.

Once Asha's baby is born, she may be able to keep the baby with her in the maternity unit, unless the baby shows signs of neonatal abstinence syndrome, in which case the baby may need to be admitted to the neonatal intensive care unit. Asha will be encouraged to breast-feed the baby as the small amount of methadone that is secreted in the breast milk will help reduce the severity of the symptoms of neonatal abstinence syndrome. Asha's interactions with the baby will be assessed while she is caring for the baby to build up a picture of her parenting abilities.

When considering Asha's desire to keep the baby with her, a number of factors need to be taken into account. As well as Asha's adherence to a methadone treatment programme and her interactions with the baby, her social situation must be considered. Asha is currently living in a hostel, which is not ideal accommodation for a newborn baby. It is also of concern that her partner is a drug dealer, since this can place both Asha and the baby at risk of serious harm. Depending on her parents' situation, it may be possible for the baby to live with them, with Asha having supervised access to the baby. The baby's father will also undergo assessment to consider if he poses a risk to the baby.

Substance misuse is complex because it has physical, emotional and social consequences for the woman and her baby. A co-ordinated multi-agency, multi-disciplinary approach is associated with improved outcomes for mothers and babies.

REFUGEES AND ASYLUM SEEKERS

Refugees and asylum seekers are vulnerable because of their status in society. They may be excluded or discriminated against or stigmatised. Some may have post-traumatic stress disorder because of their experiences and some may have physical damage as a result of their treatment. Depending on their status, they may be reluctant to identify themselves and access help. This leaves them vulnerable to exploitation.

CASE STUDY

Aku and her family are from Somalia. They fled the country and arrived in the United Kingdom where they applied for asylum. Their initial claim was refused and they are awaiting the outcome of an appeal. They are living in accommodation provided by a local charity. Aku is 28 weeks pregnant and says that the family are being harassed by locals who see them as scroungers. She is reluctant to leave the house alone, and this has led to her missing several antenatal appointments.

RESPONSE: SUPPORTING AKU

Aku is vulnerable because she is displaced, pregnant and homeless. She may lack an extended network of support. Her future in the United Kingdom is uncertain and she may fear returning to a country which is experiencing significant conflict. She and her family are experiencing hostility from their neighbours, which may increase their feelings of vulnerability and may increase the risk of emotional and mental health problems. Although she is entitled to maternity care, Aku may find it difficult to access care if she is unable to register with a GP, or if she is unable to access the services because of lack of transport or lack of knowledge about what is available. The dispersal policies adopted in the United Kingdom may further compromise care and outcomes as Aku and her family may be relocated at short notice.

Aku would benefit from a rights-based approach to care. Her position as an asylum seeker means that many decisions are taken on her behalf. For her maternity care, however, she should be fully involved in decision making. This could include using the services of an interpreter or advocate (Davies and Bath 2001). As well as enhancing communication between Aku and healthcare professionals, an advocate could also help Aku make informed choices about healthcare.

With Aku's consent, local community organisations could provide additional support for Aku. For example, asylum centres and organisations may be able to help her access benefits. Close working with groups providing housing for asylum seekers can help healthcare professionals keep in touch with women as they, and their families, are moved around. The involvement of local authorities and social services may be helpful in meeting the needs of Aku and her family.

Through careful assessment of her health and social needs, as well as those of her family, Aku can be helped through the process of pregnancy and the appeal (Newbigging and Thomas 2010). The support given to her could help reduce anxiety, improve her health and that of her family, and ensure that her baby is born into a stable and loving family environment. This, in turn, would reduce the potential for harm to her baby.

EMERGING THEMES

A number of themes have emerged from this chapter: vulnerability, communication, inequalities and person-centred care.

The evidence for vulnerability as a key factor in protecting and safeguarding children is overwhelming (Maternity Services Action Group 2011). Inequalities in health and social circumstances increase the risks to families. However, almost everyone has some resources on which they can draw, and building on these can help women and families begin to develop strategies to deal with the challenges. Underpinning effective maternity care is the concept of person-centred care. This approach empowers women and families and ensures that care is appropriate in meeting their needs, thus enhancing the outcomes for babies and children.

CONCLUSION

This chapter has addressed the principles underpinning an approach to child protection from the perspective of vulnerability. This model enables health and social care professionals to work with women and families to address issues that impact on their health and well-being and to build on strengths to increase their ability to cope with daily life and reduce the potential for child abuse.

The case studies demonstrate the range of experiences that maternity care professionals may encounter, along with possible approaches that may be taken to enhance outcomes for families. Multi-agency and inter-professional working can ensure a coherent family-centred approach to care which benefits families. Further research is needed to explore the effectiveness of vulnerability-based approaches to preventing and addressing child abuse during pregnancy and the early years period.

FURTHER READING

Lawhon, G. (2002) Facilitation of parenting the premature infant within the newborn intensive care unit. *Journal of Perinatal and Neonatal Nursing* 16(1): 71–82.
Lewis, G. (2011) Centre for maternal and child enquiries: Saving mothers' lives: Reviewing maternal deaths to make motherhood safer 2006–2008. The eighth report on confidential enquiries into maternal deaths in the United Kingdom. *BJOG* 118(Supplement 1): 1–203.20, 145–156.

REFERENCES

Afifi, T.O. and Brownridge, D.A. (2008) Physical abuse of children born to adolescent mothers: The continuation of the relationship into adult motherhood and the role of identity. In T.I. Richardson and M.V. Williams (eds), *Child Abuse and Violence*. New York: Nova Science Publishers.
Bacchus, L.J., Bewley, S., Vitolas, C.T., Aston, G., Jordan, P. and Murray, S.F. (2010) Evaluation of a domestic violence intervention in the maternity and sexual health services of a UK hospital. *Reproductive Health Matters* 18(36): 147–157.
Baker, B.L., McIntyre, L.L., Blacher, J., Cmic, K., Edelbrock, C. and Low, C. (2003) Pre-school children with and without developmental delay: Behaviour problems and parenting stress overtime. *Journal of Intellectual Disability Research* 47: 217–230.
Berrington, A., Diamond, I., Ingham, R., Stevenson, J., Borgonni, R., Hernández, C., Isabel, M. and Smith, P.W.F. (2005) Consequences of teenage parenthood: Pathways which minimise the long term negative impacts of teenage childbearing. Monograph. University of Southampton.
Botting, B., Rosato, M. and Wood, R. (1998) Teenage mothers and the health of their children. *Population Trends* 93: 19–28.
Brandon, M., Belderson, P., Warren, C., Howie, D., Gardner, R., Dodsworth, J. and Black, J. (2008) Analysing child deaths and serious injury through abuse and neglect: What can

we learn? A biennial analysis of serious case reviews 2003–5. London: Department for Children, Schools and Families.

Brett, J., Staniszewska, S., Newborn, M., Jones, N. and Taylor, L. (2011) A systematic mapping review of effective interventions for communicating with, supporting and providing information to parents of preterm infants. *BMJ Open* 1:1:e000023.

Bronte-Tinkew, J., Burkhauser, M.A. and Metz, A. (2008) *Promising Teen Fatherhood Programs*. Washington, DC: US Department of Health and Human Services.

Bryers, R. and van Teijlingen, E. (2010) Risk, theory, social and medical models: A critical analysis of the concept of risk in maternity care. *Midwifery* 6(5): 488–496.

Bunting, L. and McAuley, C. (2004) Teenage pregnancy and motherhood: The contribution of support. *Child and Family Social Work* 9(2): 207–215.

Carnevale, F.A. (2007) Revisiting Goffman's stigma: The social experience of families with children requiring mechanical ventilation at home. *Journal of Child Health Care* 11: 7–18.

Cater, S. and Coleman, L. (2006) *Planned Teenage Pregnancy: Perspectives of Young Parents from Disadvantaged Backgrounds*. York: Joseph Rowntree Foundation.

Chadwick, D.L. (2006) The evidence base in child protection. *British Medical Journal* 33: 160–161.

Chambers, R. (1989) Vulnerability, coping and policy. *IDS Bulletin* 20: 2.

Chapman, T. (2002) Safeguarding the welfare of children: 1. *British Journal of Midwifery* 10(9): 569–572.

Cloutier, P., Manion, I., Gordon-Walker, J. and Johnson, S. M. (2002) Emotionally focused interventions for couples with chronically ill children: A two-year follow-up. *Journal of Marital and Family Therapy* 28: 391–399.

Collingwood Bakeo, A. and Clarke, L. (2006) Risk factors for low birthweight on birth registration and census information, England and Wales, 1981–2000. *Health Statistics Quarterly* 30: 15–21.

Confidential Enquiry into Maternal and Child Health (CEMACH) (2011) *Perinatal Mortality 2007*. London: CEMACH.

Corlyon, J. and Stock, L. (2011) *Teenage Parenting Reference Manual*. London: Tavistock Institute of Human Relations.

Cuthbert, C., Rayns, G. and Stanley, N. (2011) *All Babies Count: Prevention and Protection for Vulnerable Babies*. London: NSPCC.

Davidson, L., King, V., Garcia, J. and Marchant, S. (2000)*Reducing Domestic Violence ... What Works? Health Services*. Home Office Briefing Note. London: Home Office.

Davies, M.M. and Bath, P.A. (2001) The maternity information concerns of Somali women in the United Kingdom. *Journal of Advanced Nursing* 36(2): 237–245.

Deave, T., Heron, J., Evan. J. and Emond, A. (2008) The impact of maternal depression in pregnancy on early childhood development. *BJOG* 115(8): 1043–1051.

Dennison, C. (2004) *Teenage Pregnancy: An Overview of the Research Evidence*. London: Health Development Agency.

Department of Health (2008) *Teenage Parents: Who Cares? A Guide to Commissioning and Delivering Maternity Services for Young Parents*. London: Department of Health.

Downe, S. (2010) Toward salutogenic birth in the 21st century. In D. Walsh and S. Downe (eds), *Essential Skills For Intrapartum Care*. Oxford: Wiley Blackwell.

Dunn, M.G., Tarter, R.E., Mezzich, A.C., Vanyukov, M., Kirisci, L. and Kirillova, G. (2002) Origins and consequences of child neglect in substance abuse families. *Clinical Psychology* 22(7): 1063–1090.

Ellefsen, B. (2002) The experience of collaboration: A comparison of health visiting in Scotland and Norway. *International Nursing Review* 49(3): 144–153.

Feldman, R., Weller, A., Sirota, L. and Eidelman, A.I. (2003) Testing a family intervention hypothesis: The contribution of mother-infant skin-to-skin contact (kangaroo care) to family interaction, proximity, and touch. *Journal of Family Psychology* 17(1): 94–107.

Fenwick, J., Barclay, L., Schmied, V. (2001) 'Chatting': an important clinical tool in facilitating mothering in neonatal nurseries. *Journal of Advanced Nursing* 33(5): 583–593.

Flach, C., Leese, M., Heron, J., Evans, J., Feder, G., Sharp, D. and Howard, L.M. (2011) Antenatal domestic violence, maternal mental health and subsequent child behaviour: A cohort study. *BJOG* 118(11): 1383–1391.

Gee, C.B. and Rhodes, J.E. (2003) Adolescent mothers' relationship with their children's biological fathers: Social support, social strain, and relationship continuity. *Journal of Family Psychology* 17(3): 370–383.

Gorin, S. (2004) *Understanding What Children Stay About Living With Domestic Violence, Parental Substance Misuse or Parental Mental Health Problems*. York: Joseph Rowntree Foundation.

Greenough, A., Cox, A., Alexander, J., Lenney, W., Turnbull, F., Burgess, S., Chetcuti, P.A.J., Shaw, N.J., Woods, A., Boorman, J., Coles, S. and Turner, J. (2001) Health care utilisation of infants with chronic lung disease, related to hospitalisation for RSV infection. *Archives of Disease in Childhood* 85(6): 463–468.

Griggs, J. and Walker, R. (2008) *The Costs of Child Poverty for Individuals and Society: A Literature Review*. York: Joseph Rowntree Foundation.

Hall, J.L. and van Teijlingen, E.A. (2006) A qualitative study of an integrated maternity, drugs and social care service for drug-using women. *BMC Pregnancy and Childbirth* 6:19.

Hamlyn, B., Brooker, S., Oleinikova, K. and Wands, S. (2002) *Infant Feeding 2000. A Survey Conducted on Behalf of the Department of Health, the Scottish Executive, the National Assembly of Wales and the Department of Health Social Services and Public Safety in Northern Ireland*. London: Stationery Office.

Harden, A., Brunton, G., Fletcher, A. and Oakley, A. (2009) Teenage pregnancy and social disadvantage: Systematic review integrating controlled trials and qualitative studies. *British Medical Journal* 339(121): b4254.

Hassall, R., Rose, J. and McDonald, J. (2005) Parenting stress in mothers of children with an intellectual disability: The effects of parental cognitions in relation to child characteristics and family support. *Journal of Intellectual Disability Research*, 11: 31–46.

Haydon, D. (2003) *Teenage Pregnancy and Looked After Children/Care Leavers: Resource for Teenage Pregnancy Co-ordinators*. London: Barnardo's.

Hodek, J., von der Schulenburg, J. and Mittendorf, T. (2011) Measuring economic consequences of preterm birth – methodological recommendations for the evaluation of personal burden on children and their caregivers. *Health Economics Review* 1: 6.

Holt, V.L., Kernic, M.A., Lumley, T., Wolf, M.E. and Rivara, F.P. (2002) Civil protection orders and risk of subsequent police-reported violence. *Journal of the American Medical Association* 288: 589–594.

Johanson, R., Newburn, M. and Macfarlane, A. (2002) Has the medicalisation of childbirth gone too far? *British Medical Journal* 324(1342): 892–895.

Jolly, M.C., Sebire, N., Harris., Robinson, S. and Regan, L. (2000) Obsteric risks of pregnancy in women less than 18 years old. *Obstetrics and Gynecology* 96(6): 962–966.

Jotzo, M. and Poets, C.F. (2005) Helping parents cope with the trauma of premature birth: An evaluation of a trauma-preventive psychological intervention. *Pediatrics* 115(4): 915–919.

Keys, M. (2005) Child protection training for primary health care teams: Making a difference? *Child Abuse Review* 14(5): 331–346.

Laming, Lord (2009) *The Protection of Children in England*. London: The Stationery Office.

Leggate, J. (2008) Improving pregnancy outcomes: Mothers and substance misuse. *British Journal of Midwifery* 16(3): 160–165.

Lewis, G. (2007) *The Confidential Enquiry into Maternal and Child Health (CEMACH). Saving Mothers' Lives: Reviewing Maternal Deaths to Make Motherhood Safer 2003– 2005. The Seventh Report on Confidential Enquiries into Maternal Deaths in the United Kingdom*. London: CEMACH.

Lounds, J.J., Borkwowski, J.G. and Whitman, T.L. (2006) The potential for child neglect: The case of adolescent mothers and their children. *Child Maltreatment* 11(3) 28–294.

Mak, W.S. and Ho, S.M. (2007) Caregiving perceptions of Chinese mothers of children with intellectual disability in Hong Kong. *Journal of Applied Research in Intellectual Disabilities* 2(2): 145–156.

Maternity Services Action Group (2011) *A Refreshed Framework for Maternity Care in Scotland*. Edinburgh: Scottish Government Health Department.

McDonnell, L., Seabrook, A., Braye, S., Bridgeman, J., Keating, H. and young father co-researchers (2009) *Talking Dads: Young Dads in Brighton and Hove Explore Parenthood. Social Work Research Report*. Brighton: University of Sussex.

Mezey, G., Bacchus, L., Haworth, A. and Bewley, S. (2003) Midwives' perceptions and experiences of routine enquiry for domestic violence. *BJOG* 110(8): 744–752.

Morris, J. (2003) *The Right Support: Report of the Task Force on Supporting Disabled Adults in their Parenting Role*. York: Joseph Rowntree Foundation.

Munro, E. (2011) *The Munro Review of Child Protection: A Child-centred System*. London: Department for Education.

National Collaborating Centre for Women's and Children's Health (2010) *Pregnancy and Complex Social Factors: A Model for Service Provision for Pregnant Women with Complex Social Factors*. London: Royal College of Obstetricians and Gynaecologists.

Newbigging, K. and Thomas N. (2010) *Good Practice in Social Care with Refugees and Asylum Seekers*. London: Social Care Institute for Excellence.

Newman, B.M. and Newman, P.R. (2009) *Development Through Life: A Psychosocial Approach*. Belmont, CA: Wadsworth.

Ortenstrand, A., Winblach, B., Nordstrom, G. and Waldenström, U. (2001) Early discharge of preterm infants followed by domiciliary nursing care: Parents' anxiety, assessment of infant health and breast-feeding. *Acta Paediatrica* 90: 1190–1195.

Piltz, A. and Wachtel, T. (2009) Barriers that inhibit nurses reporting suspected cases of child abuse and neglect. *Australian Journal of Advanced Nursing* 26(3): 93–100. Available at: www.ajan.com.au/vol26/26-3_Piltz.pdf (accessed 4 December 2013).

Poobalan, A.S., Aucott, L.S., Ross, L., Smith, W.C., Helms, P.J. and Williams, J.H. (2007) Effects of treating postnatal depression on mother-infant interaction and child development. *British Journal of Psychiatry* 191: 378–386.

Prentice, M. and Stainton, C. (2003) Outcomes of developmental care in an Australian NICU nursery. *Neonatal Network* 22(6) 17–23.

Price, S. (2004) Routine questioning about domestic violence in maternity settings. *Midwives* 7: 4.

Quinton, D., Pollock, S. and Anderson, P. (2002) *The Transition to Fatherhood in Young Men: Influences on Commitment. Summary of Key Findings*. Bristol: School for Policy Studies.

Raeside, L. (2003) Attitudes of staff towards mothers affected by substance abuse. *British Journal of Nursing*, 12(5): 302–10.

Redshaw, M. and Heikkila, K. (2010) *Delivered With Care: A National Survey of Women's Experience of Maternity Care*. Oxford: National Perinatal Epidemiology Unit, University of Oxford.

Reynolds, R. and Shams, M. (2005) Views on cultural barriers to caring for South Asian women. *British Journal of Midwifery* 13(4): 236–242.

Royal College of Psychiatrists (2011) *Parents as Patients: Supporting the Needs of Patients who are Parents and their Children. College Report 164.* London: Royal College of Psychiatrists.

Sabates-Wheeler, R. and Haddad, L. (2005) *Reconciling Different Concepts of Risk and Vulnerability.* Brighton: Institute of Development Studies.

Salmon, D., Murphy, S., Baird, K. and Price, S. (2006) An evaluation of the effectiveness of an education programme on the introduction of routine antenatal enquiry for domestic violence. *Midwifery* 22(1): 6–14.

Sibert, J.R., Maguire, S.A. and Kemp, A.M. (2007) How good is the evidence available in child protection? *Archives of Disease in Childhood* 92: 107–108.

Sidebotham, P. and the ALSPAC Study Team (2006) Patterns of child abuse in early childhood, a cohort study of the 'children of the nineties'. *Child Abuse Review* 9311–320.

Stahl, K. and Hundley, V. (2003) Risk and risk assessment in pregnancy: Do we scare because we care? *Midwifery* 19(4): 298–309.

Straus, L., McEwen, A. and Hussein, F.M. (2009) Somali women's experience of childbirth in the UK: Perspectives from Somali health workers. *Midwifery* 25(2): 181–186.

Sullivan, C. M. and Bybee, D. I. (1999) Reducing violence using community-based advocacy for women with abusive partners. *Journal of Consulting and Clinical Psychology* 67: 43–53.

Thornberry, T.P., Freeman-Gallant, A. and Lovegrove, P.J. (2009) Intergenerational linkages in antisocial behaviour. *Criminal Behaviour and Mental Health* 19(2): 80–93.

Tsianakas, V. and Liamputtong, P. (2002) What women from an Islamic background in Australia say about care in pregnancy and prenatal testing. *Midwifery* 18(1): 25–34.

van Teijlingen, E. (2005) A critical analysis of the medical model used in the study of pregnancy and childbirth. *Sociological Research Online* 10: 2.

Ward, C. and Mitchell, A. (2004) The experience of early motherhood – implications for care. *Evidence Based Medicine* 2(1): 15–27.

Wellings, K. (2001) *Country Report for Great Britain: Teenage Sexual and Reproductive Behaviour in Developed Countries. Occasional Report 6.* New York: Alan Gutmacher Institute.

Wielenga, S.M., Smith, B.J., Merkus, M.P. and Kok, J.H. (2000) Individualised developmental care in a Dutch NICU short-term clinical outcome. *Pediatrics* 105(1): 66–72.

Wiemann, C.M, Agurcia, C.A., Berenson, A.B., Volk, R.J. and Rickert, V.I. (2000) Pregnant adolescents: Experiences and behaviors associated with physical assault by an intimate partner. *Maternal and Child Health Journal* 4(2): 93–101.

World Bank (2012) *Measuring Vulnerability.* Available at: http://web.worldbank.org/WBSITE/EXTERNAL/TOPICS/EXTPOVERTY/EXTPA/0,,contentMDK:20238993~menuPK:492141~pagePK:148956~piPK:216618~theSitePK:430367,00.html (accessed 29 October 2012).

6

SUPPORTING THE DEVELOPMENT OF POSITIVE PARENTING

SUSAN REDMAN, MORAG RUSH AND GILL WATSON

CHAPTER SUMMARY

Parents are the single biggest influence on a child's life. Supporting parents in their parenting role is recognised by all governments and assemblies throughout the United Kingdom as important. The focus of this chapter is the promotion of positive parenting by healthcare practitioners working with children and their families.

What is not included within this chapter, although recognised as contributing to and impacting on parenting capabilities, are the wider structural interventions used to address compromised communities through long-term social and economic disadvantage. Therefore discussions about the role of financial measures, early years education provision, employment and childcare support measures and a whole raft of other interventions operating at societal level, that may support the tasks of parenting, are not discussed here.

This chapter explores the meaning of positive parenting and how practitioners work in partnership with parents to support child welfare and well-being. Contemporary legislation and policies are addressed in brief, highlighting the fact that for the first time, parents have identified and explicit roles and responsibilities towards their children.

Supporting parenting is a significant part of the anticipatory care role of practitioners. Quality assessment approaches, underpinned by a shared philosophy of putting children first, is at the heart of practice that seeks to prevent child harm and neglect. Although the focus of this chapter is upon supporting parents, implicit in this activity is the perception of parents and children together as part of a whole at the same time as putting children first. Therefore, supporting parenting entails enabling parents to fulfil their role, enabling them to feel satisfied that they are 'good enough' parents by building self-esteem and recognising their strengths, as well as helping to identify where help is needed and ultimately achieving positive outcomes for children.

AIMS OF THIS CHAPTER

This chapter has two aims. The first is to identify and discuss the place of parenting within the United Kingdom, taking into account the influence of legislation and policy. The second aim is to examine how practitioners can facilitate positive parenting through the application of anticipatory care in practice.

Learning outcomes

By the end of this chapter and following a period of reflection the reader will be able to:

- Understand the significance of parents and parenting in the promotion of child welfare and well-being.
- Develop awareness of positive parenting strategies, including specific parenting programmes.
- Discuss the significance of assessing risk and need in the lives of children and their parents.
- Critically analyse the knowledge and skills practitioners need to support positive parenting.

Key words

anticipatory care; assessment; intervention; positive parenting; promotion of child welfare and well-being;

Parenting is something we have all had experience of, either as a parent or as a child. Individual experiences of the role of parenting will be quite diverse and dependent upon place in time, cultural beliefs and practices, and personal capacity.

The term 'parenting' no longer applies exclusively to biological parents, with the roles and responsibilities associated with parenting falling to others, such as grandparents, other family members acting as carers, step-parents, foster and adoptive parents. Children who are 'looked after' and therefore in the care of local authorities are also cared for by others who fulfil the same roles and responsibilities as parents.

There is agreement from theorists, researchers, policy developers, parents and children that parenting matters. Parenting has a significant impact upon each one of us, the communities we live in and upon society as a whole. How we carry out parenting roles and responsibilities is therefore important. Nurturing children and young people through positive parenting is recognised as having a positive impact on their future health and mental well-being (Geddes et al. 2010).

Positive parenting is described as a parenting method which encourages better behaviour from a child. This method involves demonstrating love and affection; setting clear boundaries around expected child behaviours; praising good behaviours; listening to the child; and problem solving with the child. Positive parenting methods do not encourage physical punishments or shouting but highlight the need to address poor child behaviours through other non-physical means (NSPCC 2013).

Parents and their capacity to care for their child in a sensitive manner are of great importance. Acknowledgement of their significant role is stated within the United Nations Convention on the Rights of the Child (UNCRC) (United Nations 1989). The same Convention identifies the need for governments to support parents to carry out their parenting roles and responsibilities in caring for their children.

Children growing up within a family exposed to socioeconomic disadvantage who have the security of a loving and nurturing attachment relationship with their parents or caregivers are more likely to develop resilience to challenges experienced later in life (Children's Society 2012).

LEGISLATION AND POLICY

Up until the end of the last century and into the beginning of this century, children in the United Kingdom have been positioned by policy makers as the property of parents, without the same rights to protection from harm as adults. More recent legislative and policy changes have altered the manner in which children are cared for and protected. Chapter 1, Policy to Practice, provides a full account of both contemporary legislation and policy regarding the welfare and well-being of children across the United Kingdom.

One aspect of child welfare not fully addressed through legislation and policy is the place of physical discipline such as smacking. To date, while supporting positive parenting, none of the parliaments and assemblies within the United Kingdom have outlawed smacking through the Children Act (Department for Education and Skills 2004) and the Criminal Justice (Scotland) Act (Scottish Executive 2003). This creates a situation where what constitutes an assault against an adult cannot be applied to a child.

In a study which explored how newspapers, between the years 1989 and 2004, represented the use of smacking by parents, Redman and Taylor discovered a fundamental difference in the social positioning of children in the earliest narratives compared with more recent ones. In the earliest print media narratives, the rhetoric of parents and journalists emphasised parental control of children, while the more recent narratives recognise children's rights (Redman and Taylor 2006). The impetus of *Every Child Matters* (Department for Education and Skills 2003), *Children and Young People: From Rights to Action* (Welsh Assembly Government 2004) and *Getting it Right for Every Child* (Scottish Executive 2005) and equivalents may powerfully effect radical and far-reaching cultural change in the way that children are positioned in United Kingdom society (James and James 2004). Furthermore, there has been limited acknowledgement in real terms of children's capacity for agency; for example, their ability to participate in decision making that affects them (Alanen 2010; Bjerke 2011). However, within the recently published government policy, *Working Together to Safeguard Children* (Department for Education 2013), all adults involved in safeguarding children are challenged to act upon children's views about their need to be treated with the expectation that they are competent rather than not, and their need to be involved in and informed about the outcome of assessments and decision making.

Parents' roles and responsibilities towards their children are now recognised in legislation pertaining to children. In order to support parents in meeting their obligatory roles and responsibilities, parents have been awarded rights. These rights are only available to parents who care for a child or young person. Health and social care policies from across the United Kingdom recognise the need to share information with parents caring for children and young people.

PARENTING STRATEGIES

In line with the principles of anticipatory care, the main focus of national parenting strategies is on early intervention and prevention with an emphasis on the need for practitioners to work in partnership with parents. The Scottish Government (2012b) published a *National Parenting Strategy* which drew upon the views of parents and practitioners to bring together wide-ranging commitments that aim to support parenting. The approach taken within this strategy positions parents as part of the solution rather than focusing upon parents as part of the problem. In other words, emphasis is placed upon the identification of an individual parent's assets.

Although at the time of writing there is no equivalent comprehensive parenting support strategy for England, similar sentiments are expressed in *Parenting and Family Support: Guidance for Local Authorities* (DCSF 2010). As a result of this and similar previous guidance, in England local authorities have developed parenting strategies applicable to the communities they serve. While this may be regarded as a strength, in-keeping with current Westminster government philosophy regarding localisation, there is also a concern that without an overarching parenting strategy for England, the efforts of local authorities may be undermined, for example by competing demands on their budgets. This may result in a lack of co-ordination of efforts and is likely to result in disparity in provision across the country. Parenting UK (2012) endorsed the Scottish National Parenting Strategy, saying:

> Parenting support should not be seen only as a remedial action that is imposed when things go wrong, rather it is a preventative service which should be accessible to all.

Reflective activity

Read the job description below included in a job advertisement in a local paper:

Looking for parents to provide good care for a new baby

You will be responsible for this baby from birth until he/she is sufficiently developed and able to care for themselves. This is a 24-hour, seven days a week commitment. No authorised annual leave for years. Minimum wage with little, if any, increments for years of service. Likelihood of debt incurred.

Reflecting on your own experiences and understanding of parenting, identify what you believe to be the main activities of parenting.
You may have included some of the following:

- Keeping children safe, protecting them from harm and from danger.
- Keeping children healthy and attending to their health needs.
- Nurturing and building self-confidence by listening and by giving encouragement.
- Loving and caring; giving positive praise.
- Helping children to achieve to their full potential by enabling them to become independent.
- Supporting them with important transition times – starting Nursery/P1/High School.
- Enabling children to engage in play activity.
- Respecting children's agency or autonomy.
- Setting consistent, appropriate boundaries for behaviour.
- Enabling children to be and to feel included.
- Supporting children to make choices about things that matter to them.

The broad areas of the parenting role listed in the activity above form the basis of the outcomes for children, found within United Kingdom government policy such as *Working Together to Safeguard Children* (Department for Education 2013), *Every Child Matters* (Department for Education and Skills 2003), *Getting it Right for Every Child* (Scottish Executive 2005) and *Children and Young People: From Rights to Action* (Welsh Assembly Government 2004). These policies state what children are entitled to expect from society in terms of their rights, as well as what children and young people are expected to do (Hoyle 2008). The contribution from the Welsh Assembly Government (2004) most explicitly links specific aims and outcomes for children with sections of the United Nations Convention on the Rights of the Child (UNCRC) (United Nations 1989). The World Health Organization (2007), like the UNCRC, regards positive parenting as every child's basic human right:

> [F]or the full and harmonious development of his or her personality, [the child] should grow up in a family environment, in an atmosphere of happiness, love and understanding. (United Nations 1989: 3)

Since the needs of children and their rights as individuals and as a group are central to the above policies, practitioners are charged with putting children and young people at the centre of any assessment processes. This entails considering the child or young person as a whole, listening to their views and to the perspective of their parents. It is essential to develop communication systems that promote integrated working with other practitioners where necessary and to use evidence-based practices to support the different desired outcomes for children. Ultimately, the aims of policy and practice are to protect children from harm and to ensure that all outcomes for children are met.

While the child's interests are a primary concern and should remain the main focus when decisions are being made, parental needs also need to be voiced, heard and supported. This is crucial if parents are to be supported to care sensitively for their child. The impact of parenting on child welfare and development is significant. The next section examines the voices of parents as they describe what they perceive their support needs are in order to enable them to care for children.

THE PARENT'S PERSPECTIVE

In the report *Bringing up Children: Your Views* (Scottish Government 2012c), the main message from parents was their intent to do the best they could for their children, regardless of any difficult personal circumstances they were experiencing. However, parents identified a number of obstacles and made a number of suggestions about the sort of help they would like. The views of the parents participating in the Scottish Government study were also found in earlier studies within the United Kingdom such as that conducted by Miller and Sambell (2003). When asked what kind of things they would like help with, parents expressed a need for social change, such as more flexible childcare provision, but also high on the list of their priorities was financial advice.

Although parents clearly expressed different support needs, parents responding to the Scottish study identified more specific needs more closely related to child care, for example: managing children's behaviour, such as difficult eating and sleeping patterns; how to discipline children using positive parenting techniques; how to understand and support the different stages of their child's development; and how to build healthy relationships with their children. Fathers emphasised their need to be included in any dialogue about their children (Scottish Government 2012c). A number of other concerns were also identified:

- Parents said that they needed reassurance about 'what is normal' and that they appreciated when practitioners boosted their self-confidence by praising them when things were going well. This was particularly true for very young parents.
- Face-to-face interaction with practitioners was valued more greatly than provision of leaflets or direction to parenting websites.
- Fathers were concerned that although they wanted to be more involved in bringing up their children, they often felt excluded and perceived that healthcare professionals expected them to be able to cope.
- Fathers perceived that very few support groups addressed the needs of fathers.
- Parents recognised a need for anticipatory care as this could prevent challenging situations from becoming worse.
- Many parents expressed feelings of embarrassment about asking for support from practitioners for fear of being judged as unable to cope.

In short, there was agreement amongst parents that services should offer a 'family approach', taking into account the needs of all family members.

Reflective activity

Reflecting upon your own practice, when assessing family needs how do you recognise the contribution of fathers in caring for the child or children?

In the same way that parents voiced their different needs, they identified the need for more versatile approaches in the provision of support and education (Scottish Government 2012c).

In the earlier study exploring the parental perspective, Miller and Sambell (2003) constructed three models based on the way parents viewed support, which have implications for delivery of parenting education and outcomes for parents and children. These models are the dispensing model, the relating model and the reflecting model.

The dispensing model

- Emphasis is upon changing the child and therefore effective support is focused upon changing the child's behaviour.
- The child is viewed as the problem requiring expert advice.
- Parents who adopt this model of learning and support look to the practitioner for advice on changing specific situations and want to be told 'this is what you need to do'. In this way, parents develop a 'toolkit' of skills for use in particular situations.

A number of parenting programmes used within the United Kingdom include aspects of the dispensing model approach. For example, the Incredible Years Parenting Programme (Webster-Stratton 2001) uses educational resources such as web-based film clips and written materials to provide parents with a 'toolkit' for managing difficult parenting situations. Evaluation of such programmes indicates that many parents value this approach as they offer a range of solutions to managing challenging childrens' behaviour. Similarly, Triple P – Positive Parenting Programmes (Sanders et al. 2003), while facilitating the opportunity to create supportive networks of parents by using group work, aims to prevent severe emotional, behavioural and developmental problems in children by helping parents to manage and change children's behaviour.

The relating model

- In this model parents view support as assisting in their development as parents, focusing upon their needs and validating their role.
- Parents also value learning from each other.
- Whether the support is from peers or practitioners, the form that it takes crucially allows the reframing of parenting situations and allows identification of the strengths of parents as well as any challenges they encounter.

Within the relating model of parenting support, the need for practitioners to listen and to allow parents to communicate their views and to support capacity building is valued. Unlike the understanding of support within the dispensing model, the support within the relating model need not be expert led.

The reflecting model

- Parenting support fosters critical reflection and understanding of the interactional nature of parent–child relationships.
- Parents who respond to this type of approach are likely to ask 'Why has this happened?' rather than 'What can be done to change my child?'.
- Characteristics of this approach to parenting support rest in helping parents to explore their values and to make sense of their children's behaviour by situating it within context.

Although Miller and Sambell (2003) do not refer explicitly to ideas about 'recognition' and 'reciprocity' in their paper, it seems to be implied within this approach. The idea of reciprocity within social relationships recognises interdependence within relationships between parents and children and importantly recognises children as equals, as human beings, removing them from the position of subordination to adults. Where reciprocity amongst parent–child relationships is valued, it follows that children should and can participate in decision making about their everyday lives (Mayall 2000).

Reflecting upon the three models of approaches to parenting support, it seems likely that all three models are useful. However, it cannot be assumed that parents will respond to the same approach or that the same model will provide the range of support that parents state they need. Parenting needs are likely to change over time as children develop and family circumstances change.

Reflective activity

Reflecting on your interaction with parents, which model or approach to parenting support and education do you feel more comfortable with in your practice?

- What are your reasons for this preference?
- Which model or models support positive parenting?

PARENTAL WELL-BEING

The majority of children live with one or both parents, while others experience living with a step-parent. Whatever the arrangements, the care of the child remains paramount. However, the needs of parents who care for children cannot be ignored. Deficits in parental health and well-being as well as a lack of understanding of a child's developmental needs will impact negatively on the child's own welfare and well-being. It is therefore necessary that practitioners working and caring for children not only assess the needs of the child but also the needs of the wider family, including the parents. Enabling parents to carry out their parenting roles and responsibilities is a recognised right of every parent. The next section in this chapter explores the assessment process guided by contemporary social welfare policies.

ASSESSING PARENTAL NEED

A child-centred model such as that found within *Every Child Matters* (Department for Education and Skills 2003), *Getting it Right for Every Child* (Scottish Executive 2005), *Children and Young People Now* (Parenting UK 2012) and *Working Together to Safeguard Children* (DfE 2013) not only considers child safety, including child protection, but also addresses other health and well-being risks and needs. These additional areas encompass health, educational and social outcomes.

Parents and practitioners, working in partnership, are able to identify risks and needs for a child using an assessment based upon these outcomes. Generally, it is parents/caregivers who are expected to meet their child's needs using their parenting skills and knowledge. Whilst appreciating the resources and skills parents already use to meet these needs, a structured assessment based upon child-centred outcomes helps parents identify and plan any additional support required.

In our experience while working with NHS health visitor colleagues in Scotland, we have been able to observe first-hand how policy has been interpreted in a pragmatic way, with the development of practical assessment tools, which place children at the centre of assessment and foster capacity building and partnership working with parents. There is an expectation in *Every Child Matters* (DfES 2003) and *Getting it Right for Every Child* (Scottish Executive 2005) and the Welsh equivalent *Children and Young People: From Rights to Action* (Welsh Assembly Government 2004) that any problem identified through assessment will be contextualised within a broader picture of the child's world.

With the child at the centre with the dimensions 'How I grow and develop', 'What I need from people who look after me' and 'My world' (see Figure 6.1), practitioners are invited to view situations from a child's perspective, recognising environmental, social and economic factors which influence specific outcomes for each individual child.

This philosophy is shared within *Working Together to Safeguard Children* (Department for Education 2013), *Every Child Matters* (DfES 2003), *Getting it Right for Every Child* (Scottish Executive 2005) and *Children and Young People: From Rights to Action* (Welsh Assembly Government 2004). This child-centred philosophy is underpinned by recognition of children's rights to have their views

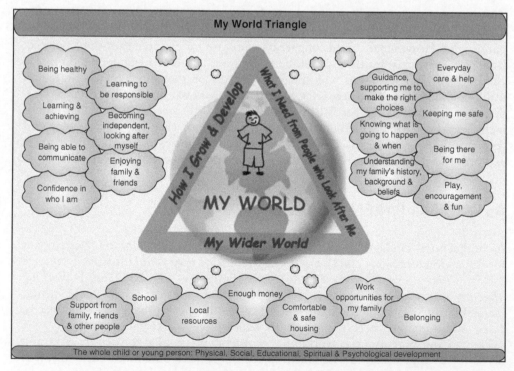

Figure 6.1 My World triangle (Department of Health 2000)

heard and to be taken into consideration when any decision is being made about their care.

The assessment framework identifies different aspects of the child's world represented by the acronyms SHEEP in *Every Child Matters* and SHANARRI in *Getting it Right for Every Child*. Each acronym provides helpful reminders of the desired outcomes for children.

Every Child Matters identifies five outcomes for children (SHEEP)

Every Child Shall be
- Safe
- Healthy
- Enjoy life/Achieve
- Enjoy Economic wellbeing
- Positive contribution in decision making

Getting it Right for Every Child identifies eight outcomes for children (SHANARRI)

Every child shall be
- Safe
- Healthy
- Achieving
- Nurtured
- Active
- Respected
- Responsible
- Included

The following case study and activity provides an opportunity to apply the assessment framework to a family situation. Take time to read through the case study carefully before doing the activity.

Gavin is a young single parent. He lives in a local authority flat in a small town and is currently unemployed. He left school with few qualifications. Gavin's relationships with his ex-partner, who is the mother of his children, and his parents have broken down. Gavin has three children, David aged 4 years, Billy aged 3 years and Mia aged

(Continued)

CASE STUDY

(Continued)

13 months. Gavin recently had a meeting with David's nursery teacher who was concerned that he had not had any breakfast before nursery and was not always properly washed and dressed for nursery. Gavin confided with the teacher that he desperately wants to be a 'good dad' but is experiencing a high level of stress and anxiety about child rearing and his personal life and relationships. Home life has become increasingly chaotic and routines have broken down. The teacher advised Gavin to make an appointment to talk things over with his health visitor (practitioner).

Activity

- You are the practitioner Gavin contacts for advice regarding his children.
- Using the outcomes for children derived from policy (e.g. SHEEP or SHANNARI or another framework that you are familiar with), identify the kinds of information you will need to collect in order that you are more able to support Gavin.

Next, read through the continuing case study in which a practitioner has made notes about her/his observations when visiting Gavin and the children. SHANARRI has been used as the framework for assessment (but you may have used SHEEP) and demonstrates how the assessment is documented. Take time to compare the practitioner's notes with your own, and identify any differences and commonalities.

CASE STUDY

Assessment of needs and risks using eight outcomes for children (SHANARRI).

Overall

Safe

The family live in a second floor, two-bedroom flat that is temporary accommodation until they are offered a permanent house by their local authority. The two older boys share a bedroom. Mia sleeps in a cot, sharing her dad's bedroom. The home has enough basic furniture to meet their needs. There are toys everywhere but the home is clean. Gavin has to buy cards to operate the gas central heating and electricity. From the living room there is access to a small veranda that has a metal fence around 1.5 metres high. This is where David tends to put the washing out to dry but otherwise it dries in the house. This can be a problem as it can take a while to dry. From the common stair there is a garden shared with the other tenants but it is not completely fenced in. An upstairs neighbour allows his dog to defecate on the grass.

Despite his self-reported high levels of stress and anxiety, Gavin's general presentation is good. He does not use substances except for cigarettes but says he does this outside on the veranda. There is no smell of tobacco/ashtrays in the home which suggests the children are not at risk of passive smoking. He engages positively in discussion and appears receptive to advice and information.

The children

Healthy

David aged 4:

- Development: achieving milestones for age.
- Overdue his vision screen by the orthoptist.
- Growth: although not measured recently he appears in proportion for height/weight. Described by his dad as a fussy eater who will not eat any fruit except bananas. Has limited variety of food groups.
- Immunisations: up to date with UK immunisation programme.
- Not registered with a dentist.
- Attended A&E last month – laceration to forehead after falling off a wall.
- Diagnosed with asthma last year and prescribed inhalers. Now overdue his review by Asthma Nurse at GP practice.

Billy aged 3:

- Development: wearing pull-ups during the day and nappies at night. Dad has tried formal toilet training but has given up again recently.
- Growth: not measured recently but appears in proportion. Dad reports he is a good eater.
- Immunisations: up to date with UK programme.
- Not registered with a dentist.

Mia aged 13 months:

- Development: not yet using a cup, still given bottles of milk/juice throughout the day. Goes to sleep at night with a bottle of milk.
- Uses a dummy throughout the day. Not yet walking independently but able to cruise furniture/pull herself up to stand.
- Growth: not measured recently but appears in proportion. Dad reports she is a good eater.
- Immunisations: now due 13-month immunisations.
- Not registered with a dentist.

Achieving

David is in his preschool year at a local authority nursery, attending five morning sessions each week. His teachers are beginning to prepare David for his transition to Primary 1. Nursery staff have noticed that when David has not had breakfast or arrives late he finds it more difficult to settle into constructive activities and tends to misbehave.

Billy is due to start Nursery at the next intake in 4 months' time.

At present neither Billy nor Mia attend any preschool groups.

(Continued)

(Continued)

Nurtured

Mia has a strong attachment to Gavin who has been her main carer since she was 6 weeks old. Gavin is responsive to Mia's need for attention, giving her reassurance and cuddles appropriately. Gavin appears calm and relaxed when he is holding her. They interact well together and enjoy play activities. Mia responds to Gavin with lots of chatter and smiles.

The boys have had difficulty adjusting to their mother not being around. Gavin is aware of this and feels guilty about it. Gavin finds it more difficult to relate with the boys in a more constructive way. The boys' behaviour stresses him and sometimes makes him angry. They ignore instructions not to climb on the furniture or eat their meals and are openly defiant when he gives them a row by mimicking his responses. He shouts at them for minor misbehaviours such as attention seeking whilst he is on his mobile. He is constantly saying 'no' to them. The angrier he gets, the more cheeky the boys become.

Gavin has vocalised to David's nursery teacher that he is feeling stressed and anxious. On further discussion with the practitioner he is keen to discuss his feelings further.

Active

The children enjoy playing outside and Gavin tries to take them to a nearby park when he can. He finds it difficult to keep control of the boys and at the same time push Mia's buggy when out and about. Billy has no road sense and likes to run when he gets any opportunity.

There is a local community centre and a library but Gavin has not had the confidence to go and see if there are appropriate activities for the children as he is worried that it might cost him money.

Respect and Responsibility

The lack of good daily routines and inconsistent boundary setting mean that the boys tend not to listen to Gavin's instructions. The boys do not respond when he shouts. The boys jump on the beds, sofa and chairs, which Gavin either ignores or gets very stressed about. Toys are broken regularly and there are now no books as they have had all their pages ripped out.

Included

Gavin makes all the decisions in relation to meeting the children's health and well-being needs. As the children mature they need to learn to make decisions and be given choices about the things in their lives that impact and matter to them.

The practitioner has recorded the details of all three children as well as Gavin, taking note of the home environment and that of the close amenities available to the family. The detail is helpful in identifying the level of health and well-being for

Table 6.1 Assessment of risks/needs and required actions to address risks/needs (following the SHANARRI framework)

Outcome	Risks/Needs	Possible Action/s
Safe	• The family requires a 3-bedroom property, as they are currently overcrowded. • The common stair and garden need to be maintained to an acceptable standard to allow the children easy access to a clean and safe outdoor area where they can learn through outdoor play activities. • The windows need to have childproof locks. • The children need to be supervised closely when the door to the veranda is unlocked/open. • The home environment needs to be kept warm and comfortable.	• PRACTITIONER/Gavin to complete referral for housing support in local area. • PRACTITIONER/Gavin to complete referral to local community safety project. • Gavin to ensure the children are supervised at all times. • Gavin to make an appointment with local citizens' advice service to check his benefit entitlement. • Gavin to consider attending household budgeting sessions being run at local Family Centre.
Healthy	• The children need to attend all their medical appointments. • Growth and development need to be monitored as per UK Healthy Child programme (Scottish Government 2011). • The children need to be registered with a dentist and have regular dental check ups. • Father needs some support with understanding and encouraging age appropriate developmental milestones – toilet training, eating, self-soothing.	• Gavin to make appointments for the outstanding immunisations/medical reviews at GP practice. • Gavin to ensure the children attend all scheduled growth/development reviews. • Gavin to register the children with a local dentist. • PRACTITIONER to offer one-to-one general parenting support using an approach that builds upon Gavin's assets, such as the Solihull approach. • PRACTITIONER/Gavin to complete referral to local family centre for next available group parenting support programme.
Achieving	• The boys need a stable home environment that will help them get the most out of any formal learning opportunities. • The children require a daily routine that allows them to engage effectively in their learning. • Mia and Billy could benefit socially and educationally from the opportunity to attend a structured preschool environment.	• PRACTITIONER/Gavin to complete referral for family worker support through local nursery/family centre to help establish daily routines. • Gavin to ensure David attends all nursery sessions. • Gavin to consider applying for a place at a local playgroup for Billy. • Gavin to consider attending a local parent/toddler group with the younger children.

(Continued)

Table 6.1 (Continued)

Outcome	Risks/Needs	Possible Action/s
Nurtured	• All of the children need a loving and reciprocal relationship with their father. • Gavin's poor mental health (stress and anxiety) may negatively impact on the children's emotional development. • The children need Gavin to be available emotionally for them. Gavin needs to consider and understand his own feelings so that he can then deal with the children's feelings and behaviour.	• PRACTITIONER/Gavin to consider appropriate mental health assessment and support for Gavin. • Gavin to consider the support of a Home-Start (UK charitable organisation offering parent support) volunteer. • Gavin to consider referral to a local Dad's Group for peer and professional support.
Active	• The children need to be aware of road safety. • The boys need to have constructive activities that promote their general development and use up their energy. • Gavin needs to be enabled to develop confidence in his parenting skills.	• Gavin to consider support getting out and about safely in the community – this could be a focus for the Home-Start volunteer. • Gavin to consider referral to a local Dad's Group where they offer a parenting support programme and other activities tailored for fathers.
Respected/ Responsible	• There is a risk that Gavin may resort to inappropriate ways of dealing with the boys e.g. smacking. • The boys need the security of consistent boundary setting by Gavin so that they understand what behaviour is expected of them. • The boys need to have a daily routine where they know what is happening next. • The children need to learn to look after their toys and family possessions.	• Gavin to consider whether support and encouragement with positive parenting strategies could be a focus for the allocated family worker. • Healthcare team to reinforce and encourage any of Gavin's new learning with other agencies.
Included	• As the children mature they need to learn to make decisions and be given choices about the things in their lives that impact and matter to them.	• When developmentally appropriate Gavin to offer the children simple choices in their daily activities e.g. food, clothing, games and books.

each family member. It is clear that in the main each child appears to be developing within the expected boundaries for their developmental age. The immediate home environment appears safe but the environment external to the home is less so because of the lack of a safe and secure play area.

Gavin appears to have the children's best interests under his consideration. The fact that the children appear to be reaching the physical, social and psychological developmental goals is an asset and reflects fulfilment of his roles and responsibilities. However, there are some signs that not all the children's health needs are being addressed, as highlighted by the lack of dental care and missing out immunisations. Gavin may also require support to identify locations where his children can play in a safe and secure environment. This is not always easy as all three of Gavin's children are at differing stages of development. As identified, Gavin is receptive to information and advice.

To be of value and to have a functional use, the assessment of Gavin and his family needs to be organised and presented to identify risks or needs together with the proposed action to address the same risk or need. By identifying action points, it is then possible to enable progress, or even deterioration, to be measured, monitored and addressed if required. Evaluation of the family must be undertaken to ensure that progress is made.

Table 6.1 presents the findings of each of the assessment activities and action points pertaining to the assessment of Gavin and his children. The noted action points need to be developed by Gavin and the practitioner together, and in partnership. The responsibility for addressing each point is then transparent and acknowledged.

PLANNING AND ACTION

The above assessment is helpful in establishing what is known about the health and well-being of Gavin's children and perceptions about Gavin's capacity for parenting. An analysis of the assessment results in the identification of possible or potential courses of action that need to be prioritised in partnership with the family. Interventions from other universal services, as well as the inclusion of third sector agencies, may be considered appropriate as a means of supporting Gavin to care for his children.

It is helpful at this stage to identify how organisations, through their practitioners, can work with parents to meet their needs as well as meeting the needs of their children. A shared assessment framework and plan for action allows other support agencies to easily identify and build on the support the practitioner is providing. In partnership with other supporting agencies (e.g. social services, Nursery, Home-Start, Gingerbread), practitioners are required to set a date for reviewing the effectiveness of any intervention and to allow parents to reflect upon action and achievements. This may be followed by setting new goals.

Partnership working with parents and children involves gaining an understanding of their personal strengths and limitations and their expectations of themselves.

In the example of Gavin's family, it may have occured to you that their strengths were not included in the assessment process. Parents and children's strengths can be regarded as 'resilience factors' or, to use a more everyday term, their 'assets'. The idea of assets includes personal qualities as well as external supports, such as having positive close family ties or engagement in community activities.

PARENTING PROGRAMMES SUPPORTING POSITIVE PARENTING

There are a wide variety of supports for meeting the needs of parents and their families. The vast majority work with parents to address their needs in order that parents are better prepared to safeguard their children sensitively and appropriately.

There are a number of parenting programmes in the United Kingdom which recognise the need to acknowledge family assets and thereby to empower and motivate parents to practice sensitive parenting. For example, the Mellow Parenting Programme (Mills and Puckering 1995). The programme's central aim is to empower parents by fostering reflexivity. Parents are encouraged to make connections between the effects of their own past and present experiences on their behaviour towards their children. One way to achieve this is to ask parents to relate a little of their own growing-up experiences; to tell their own story. Practitioners who use biographical narrative have found it to be a powerful tool that can help the narrator to make connections between their own experience of being a child and how they perceive their current parenting role. Another example of how biographical narrative may be used when working with parents can be found within the Solihull Parenting Programme. This is an approach and a resource developed for use by care professionals working with families, babies, children and young people who are affected by emotional and behavioural difficulties (Solihull NHS Care Trust 2006).

The imperative to build parenting capacity by identifying parental assets underpins the Parents Altogether Lending Support (PALS) programme (Zeedyk et al. 2002). PALS consists of a series of parenting groups in which, although facilitated by trained counsellors, value is placed upon the experiences of group members. The group approach fosters the development of supportive networks of parents. The overall aim of PALS is to help parents to gain confidence and to practice parenting skills through problem solving, which in turn raises self-esteem (Moran et al. 2004).

ASSESSMENT OF RISK

A formal assessment of risk or need is the starting point before any programme or interventions can begin. There has to be alignment between the identified risk or risks and the introduction of appropriate interventions which best suits the child, family and their situation. While frameworks guide the assessment process, it is the capabilities of the practitioner which contribute substantially to the overall quality of the assessment, as discussed in Chapter 4. Capabilities in this chapter refer to the integration of knowledge, critical thinking skills and psychological awareness and empathy. The next section briefly examines the role of the knowledge and skills necessary to assess the needs of children and parents.

KNOWLEDGE AND SKILLS REQUIRED BY PRACTITIONERS

Reflecting upon the case study of Gavin's family, a range of knowledge and skills are required to enable a rigorous assessment of health needs and delivery of evidence-based intervention, in partnership with children, young people and families. The main kinds of knowledge and skills required to assess children and their parents are listed below.

Knowledge and skills for professionals working with children and parents

Here are examples of the knowledge, skills and professional standards required by practitioners working in partnership with and assessing the needs of children and their families.
- Knowledge and understanding of:

  o child development
  o attachment relationships
  o overarching theories and approaches that inform practice, e.g. critical thinking including reflection and reflexivity
  o protective factors and resilience
  o parental capacity
  o evidence-based interventions
  o other services
  o local policies and pathways of care.

- Skills:

  o communication
  o networking
  o ability to work in partnership.

- Professional standards:

  o accountability
  o responsibility
  o access to robust supervision.

This is not a definitive list of knowledge, skills and standards.

The suggestions listed above mirror the knowledge, skills and values for parenting support by children's workforces, including universal services and the third sector, identified by the Scottish Government (2012a) and the Department for Education (2013).

Across different agencies the core knowledge, skills and values are the same; however, the level of each will depend on the role. For example, the knowledge and skills expected from a community nurse will be at a different level from that of a parent volunteer working in a family centre. Similar aspects of knowledge and skills are identified within equivalent guidance published by the Welsh Assembly Government (2004) and the Department for Children, Schools and Families (2010). Implications for such knowledge and skills frameworks for parenting support include the need for service managers to ensure that everyone involved in working with children, young people and families participates in appropriate education and training and to invest in management systems that support regular quality supervision of practitioners.

EMERGING THEMES

Practitioners working with children and their families have a significant role in supporting positive parenting to maximise physical, social and psychological outcomes for children. A structured and sensitive approach to assessment will help to identify the kinds of support parents need in order to fulfil their roles and responsibilities.

Parenting support is anticipatory in nature and asset-based, and is aligned with a public health approach to safeguarding children and young people. In other words, parenting support is concerned with prevention of harm, physical and emotional, by anticipating the needs of children and parents. It is underpinned by the idea of relationships: ways of working in partnership with parents to foster child–parent relationships that are characterised by mutuality, reciprocity and respect, ultimately contributing to the development of children's agency.

CONCLUSION

In this chapter parenting support needs have been explored in the context of current policy that places children's needs at the centre. Practitioners promoting positive parenting must consider the needs of the whole family, identifying assets as well as any challenges in their ability to ensure positive outcomes for their children. Partnership working with the family and support agencies using shared frameworks for assessment and planning assist in identifying timely interventions that safeguard child health and well-being. Practitioners can facilitate positive parenting by adopting problem solving approaches and by helping parents to recognise and respect children's rights through encouraging families to develop reciprocity in parent and child relationships.

A range of parenting support approaches have been considered that can help practitioners and families to achieve their goals towards good-enough parenting and secure, happy children who will become confident, caring young people and adults.

FURTHER READING

Geddes, R., Haw, S. and Frank, J. (2010) *Interventions for Promoting Early Childhood Development for Health*. Edinburgh: SCPHRP. Available at: www.scphrp.ac.uk/node/103 (accessed 20 December 2013).

NSPCC (2013) *Encouraging Better Behaviour: A Practical Guide to Positive Parenting*. Available at: www.nspcc.org.uk/help-and-advice/for-parents-and-carers/guides-for-parents/better-behaviour/better-behaviour-pdf_wdf90719.pdf (accessed 20 December 2013).

Syvertsen, A.K., Roehlkepartain, E. and Scales, P.C. (2012) *Key Findings from the American Family Assets Study*. Minneapolis, MN: Search Institute.

REFERENCES

Alanen, L. (2010) Taking children's rights seriously. *Childhood* 17(5): 5.

Bjerke, H. (2011) Children as 'differently equal' responsible beings: Norwegian children's views of responsibility. *Childhood* 18(1): 67–80.

Children's Society (2012) *The Good Childhood Report*. London: The Children's Society.

Department for Children, Schools and Families (DCSF) (2010) *Parenting and Family Support: Guidance for Local Authorities in England*. Nottingham: DCSF Publications.

Department for Education (DfE) (2013) *Working Together to Safeguard Children: A Guide to Inter-agency Working to Safeguard and Promote the Welfare of Children*. London: The Stationery Office.

Department for Education and Skills (DfES) (2003) *Every Child Matters*. London: The Stationery Office.

Department for Education and Skills (DfES) (2004) *The Children Act*. London: The Stationery Office.

Department of Health (2000) *Framework for the Assessment of Children in Need and their Families*. London: The Stationery Office. Available at: http://webarchive.nationalarchives.gov.uk/+/www.dh.gov.uk/en/publicationsandstatistics/publications/publicationspolicyandguidance/dh_4003256 (accessed 20 December 2013).

Geddes, R., Haw, S. and Frank, J. (2010) *Interventions for Promoting Early Childhood Development for Health*. Edinburgh: SCPHRP. Available at: www.scphrp.ac.uk/node/103 (accessed 20 December 2013).

Hoyle, D. (2008) 'Problematising Every Child Matters', the encyclopaedia of informal education. Available at: www.infed.org/socialwork/every_child_matters_a_critique.htm (accessed 20 December 2013).

James, A. and James, A.L. (2004) *Constructing Childhood: Theory, Policy and Social Practice*. London: Palgrave.

Mayall, B. (2000) The sociology of childhood in relation to children's rights. *Journal of Children's Rights* 8: 243–259.

Miller, S. and Sambell, K. (2003) What do parents feel they need? Implications of parents' perspectives for the facilitation for parenting programmes. *Children and Society* 17: 32–44.

Mills, M. and Puckering, C. (1995) Bringing about change in parent–child relationships, in J. Trowell and M. Bower (eds), *The Emotional Needs of Young Children and their Families: Using Psychoanalytic Ideas in the Community*. New York: Taylor and Francis/Routledge. pp. 136–147.

Moran, P., Gate, D. and van de Merwe, A. (2004) *What Works in Parenting Support: A Review of the International Evidence*. Policy Research Bureau, Department for Education and Skills. Nottingham: The Stationery Office.

NSPCC (2013) *Encouraging Better Behaviour*. Available at: www.nspcc.org.uk/help-and-advice/for-parents-and-carers/guides-for-parents/better-behaviour/better-behaviour-pdf_wdf90719.pdf (accessed 12 December 2013).

Parenting UK (2012) *Children and Young People Now*. Available at: www.cypnow.co.uk/cyp/news/1074892/england-urged-follow-scotlands-lead-extending-parenting-support (accessed 21 November 2012).

Redman, S. and Taylor, J. (2006) Legitimate family violence as represented in the print media: Textual analysis. *Journal of Advanced Nursing* 56(2): 157–165.

Sanders, M., Cann, W. and Markie-Dadds, C. (2003) The Triple P – Positive Parenting Programme: A universal population-level approach to the prevention of child abuse. *Child Abuse Review*, 12(3): 155–71.

Scottish Executive (2003) *The Criminal Justice (Scotland) Act*. Edinburgh: Scottish Executive.

Scottish Executive (2005) *Getting it Right for Every Child*. Edinburgh: Scottish Executive.

Scottish Government (2011) *A New Look at Hall 4: The Early Years. Good Health for Every Child.* Available at: www.scotland.gov.uk/Resource/Doc/337318/0110676.pdf (accessed 13 December 2013).

Scottish Government (2012a) *The Common Core Skills, Knowledge and Understanding and Values for the 'Children's Workforce' in Scotland*. Edinburgh: Scottish Government.

Scottish Government (2012b) *National Parenting Strategy: Making a Positive Difference to Children and Young People through Parenting*. Edinburgh: Scottish Government.

Scottish Government (2012c) *Bringing up Children: Your Views*. Edinburgh: Scottish Government.

Solihull NHS Care Trust (2006) *Solihull Approach Resource: The First Five Years*. Solihull: NHS Care Trust.

United Nations (1989) *United Nations Convention on the Rights of the Child*. Geneva: United Nations.

Webster-Stratton, C. (2001) The incredible years: Parents, teachers, and children training series. *Residential Treatment for Children and Youth* 18: 31–45.

Welsh Assembly Government (2004) *Children and Young People: From Rights to Action*. Cardiff: Welsh Assembly.

World Health Organization (2007) *Primary Prevention of Intimate-partner Violence and Sexual Violence: Background Paper for WHO Expert Meeting*. Available at: www.who.int/violence_injury_prevention/publications/violence/IPV-SV.pdf (accessed 31 January 2013).

Zeedyk, M.S., Werritty, I. and Riach, C. (2002) The PALS parenting support programme: Lessons learned from the evaluation of processes and outcomes. *Children and Society* 16: 318–333.

7

FAMILY-CENTRED CARE

JO CORLETT AND GILL WATSON

CHAPTER SUMMARY

Since the 1980s, paediatric nurses have favoured using nursing models or frameworks to guide care delivery for children (Casey 1993). One such model which has received much attention since those early beginnings is family-centred care (Shields 2010). According to Shields, family-centred care requires parents, and the wider family, to work in partnership with paediatric nurses to address the care, welfare, developmental and safety needs of the child. Today, family-centred care can no longer be considered a new concept as it has evolved over the years, bringing to the surface the positive nature families can have on the developing child (Brandon et al. 2011).

The practice of family-centred care has not occurred without critics and tensions. There are those who question the fit between family-centred models of care and contemporary child-centric legislation and social policies. No longer are children viewed as the 'property' of their parents but as individuals with rights of their own, to be respected by all others, including individuals, services, organisations and society (Kelly et al. 2012). While this point is pertinent in today's health and social care practices, parents cannot be ignored or left on the sidelines. Parents and families have a significant part to play in the lives of children, as made explicit by the United Nations Convention on the Rights of the Child (United Nations 1989). This point is supported through legislation where, for the first time in history, parental roles and responsibilities towards the child are made explicit. Parents therefore now have identified rights to enable them to meet their parenting roles and responsibilities, as discussed throughout this book.

Similarly, practitioners in health and social care organisations also have roles and responsibilities towards meeting the needs of children. It is possible to consider that in the majority of families, parents are capable of providing the emotional warmth and holistic encouragement that every child and young person has the right to receive. However, the notion that some families are 'low on warmth and high on criticism' (Cawson 2002) remains a real problem and possibly contributes to many psychological issues developed in childhood (Glaser 2011). Therefore there is an argument for engaging with such families, and intervening early can bring about positive outcomes (Allen 2011). Framing practice delivery to children must include a set of principles which acknowledge the significance of the family. Healthcare for children should be managed within a family-centred model because of the potential it offers in helping families to safeguard their children.

This chapter will explore the historical development of family-centred care within the United Kingdom before discussing the defining elements of the framework. An alternative definition for patient- (child-) and family-centred care is presented and discussed. To understand the tensions experienced in practice regarding family-centred care, a literature review is presented. This review informs the development of emerging themes for consideration in contemporary child and family-care practice.

AIMS OF THIS CHAPTER

This chapter has three aims. The first aim is to provide a historical review and understanding of the development of family-centred care in healthcare in the United Kingdom. The second aim is to define and discuss the main concepts of family-centred care before identifying an alternative, which offers greater alignment with the principles underpinning contemporary social welfare policies. The third aim of this chapter is to review the literature exploring the strengths and limitations of family-centred care in healthcare. This will inform emerging themes for future considerations.

Learning outcomes

After reading this chapter and following a period of reflection the reader will be able to:

- Develop an awareness of the historical events that have contributed towards the development of family-centred care.
- Critically evaluate the concept of family-centred care, identifying its strengths and limitations.
- Develop an understanding of parental roles, responsibilities and rights of parents.
- Critically analyse how the application of family-centred care in practice can support families struggling to meet the welfare and developmental needs of their child.

Key words

communication; family; family-centred care; parental roles, parents; partnership; responsibilities and rights

Family-centred care is a model of care delivery more commonly used in child health services within the Western world (Shields et al. 2006). This does not mean that such an approach is not used in under-developed countries; however, less is known about the application of family-centred practices in those countries.

According to Casey (1993), the 1980s witnessed 'model fever' gathering momentum in nurse education and latterly in clinical nursing. Family-centred care was one such model, often referred to as a 'framework' to guide the care provided by paediatric nurses to children and their families. Since those early beginnings family-centred models of care have been adopted by other nursing disciplines, midwifery and other professional groups such as social work.

Since the 1980s, the status of children in our society has evolved. The 'rights-based' agenda has framed child care and welfare legislation across the United Kingdom. No longer are children considered the 'property' of their families, rather they are equal to all others in society and need to be viewed as individuals with rights of their own. Child-centric policies are now driving child welfare and safeguarding practices. This new direction raises a number of questions about the significance and role of the family to the child.

Families are recognised as having a significant part to play in the lives of children. The United Nations Convention on the Rights of the Child (UNCRC) (United Nations 1989) supports the family environment as the best place for a child to flourish. There is a general acceptance that many parents in families with one or more children are sensitive to their child's needs and are capable of providing the emotional warmth and learning experiences to enable that child to reach their potential. Some children, however, are exposed to serious risk because of parents' poor lifestyles, relationship difficulties or mental illness, and exist in a home environment which lacks the necessary warmth, learning and developmental experiences. For children living with parents and families where substance use is common, where there is domestic violence or who have parents with unstable mental illness, the risk of exposure to long-term neglect and possible abuse is increased.

The status of children in our society has changed considerably, moving from having a lowly level of insignificance to being a citizen with identical rights to that of other humans. Reflecting on these changes brings to the fore an opportunity to review the appropriateness of using family-centred care in healthcare practice today.

HISTORICAL DEVELOPMENT

Prior to World War II, healthcare professionals cared for the child in hospital, with minimal involvement of parents and the wider family. Attitudes towards healthcare provision for children began to change post-war as the effects of long-term separation of children from their families, necessitated by the mass evacuation of children from urban areas, began to emerge (Shields 2010). Shields cites the early research carried out by Anna Freud, daughter of Sigmund Freud, who discovered that children injured during bombing raids were more likely to maintain their psychological health if they remained with their mothers. Work by other researchers also demonstrated that children hospitalised in various contexts were more psychologically and emotionally resilient than those separated from their parents. Whilst this early work served to highlight the potential effects of separating ill children from their families, it was two British researchers, John Bowlby and James Robertson, who were the principal instigators of what would become the family-centred approach to child healthcare provision (Shields 2010).

John Bowlby, a child psychiatrist and pioneer of attachment theory, provided the means of understanding and explaining the emotional impact, expressed through grief and anxiety, that a young child experiences when separated from their mother (Bowlby 1944a; 1944b). James Robertson, a social worker, used Bowlby's theory to examine the effects of child–mother separation as a result of hospitalisation of the child (Jolley and Shields 2009). The work of these and other early researchers resulted in the production of the Platt Report (Ministry of Health 1959), commissioned by the British government, and was subsequently the catalyst to change the provision of paediatric services worldwide. However, family-centred care did not immediately emerge as the fully formed concept it is today, rather it has matured gradually as the benefits of including parents and families in caring for the child have become apparent. This is evident in various terms that have been used over the last 50 years to describe this developing concept. These terms have ranged from parental participation, care-by-parent, parental involvement, negotiated care, partnership-in-care and family-centred care, reflecting the gradual shift in emphasis on care provided for the child by the health professional to care provided for and with the family.

MODELS OF CARE WITHIN THE CONTEXT OF CONTEMPORARY SOCIAL POLICY

Contemporary policies across the United Kingdom recognise that all universal services coming into contact with children, directly or indirectly, apply a child-focused model to guide practice: *Every Child Matters* in England (Department of Education and Skills. 2003), *Getting it Right for Every Child* in Scotland (Scottish Executive 2005), *Children and Young People: From Rights to Action* in Wales (Welsh Assembly Government 2004) and *Our Children and Young People – Our Shared Responsibility: The Reform Implementation Process in Child Protection Services in Northern Ireland* (Northern Ireland Assembly 2006). This is a major step forward and remains at the forefront of care and interventions for any child living within or outwith a family context. However, as noted by Hall et al.

(2010), policies informing children's services within the United Kingdom have located children and families in separate worlds, isolating children from the context of their families. While there is a need to emphasise the significance of the best interests of the child when considering and making decisions regarding child development, welfare and protection, these same elements more often than not are delivered within the family context.

The UNCRC (United Nations 1989) views the family as crucial to the developing child, so much so that eight of the 54 Articles contained within the Convention provide guidance on parental involvement relating to the rights of children. The UNCRC also highlights the responsibilities of government to support families to meet the needs of their children. While the Convention is not legislation in itself, it is a legal instrument with the power to influence national legislation as well as social and health policies developed to meet the needs of the population.

Legislation across all four nations identified the roles and responsibilities of parents towards their children, and to meet their responsibilities parents have rights. Parental rights referred to within Scottish legislation, with similar definitions across the other nations within the United Kingdom, are privileged rights, existing only to enable parents to fulfil parental responsibilities towards their children to

> safeguard and promote the child's health, development and welfare; to provide direction and guidance in a manner appropriate to the child's stage of development. (Sutherland 2001: 93)

This statement makes explicit the responsibilities of parents towards meeting the needs of children. Every parental decision taken to address a child's needs must be made in the best interests of the child. It is therefore important in healthcare when caring for children to be aware of parental rights in order to support parents to meet their responsibilities towards their child's developmental, welfare and health needs. Across all universal services but in particular in healthcare delivery there is a need and great opportunity to work with parents to address what must be considered the best interests of the child. Family-centred care provides a model of care to support children within the context of their families.

Parents and the wider family who are sensitive as well as responsive to the developmental needs of the child are more likely to provide a suitable physical, emotional and social environment from which the child can grow and develop (Britto and Ulkuer 2012). The overall quality of the home environment created by parents shapes the day-to-day parent–child interactions. Family orientated child experiences, both in and outwith the home, address health and safety issues such as nutrition, immunisation, protection from accidents and violence (Guralnick 2009).

While the quality of the child–parent relationship and subsequent interaction is strongly guided by psycho-social attachment patterns and influenced by ecological elements, the family is recognised as playing a central part in addressing the rights of the child. Yet while contemporary policy identifies parents as significant to the child, either in a positive of negative context, there is no comprehensive framework for practitioners to use to engage with parents. It is the engaging, relational and participatory processes inherent within family-centred care that best support engagement with parents to meet the needs of the child.

Fully implemented family-centred care is considered of benefit to healthcare practitioners, parents, family members and most importantly the child (Shields et al. 2006). The implementation of this guiding framework now extends beyond the hospital setting, stretching into every context in which a child's health and social needs are considered and addressed (Franck and Callery 2004). Family-centred care enables healthcare providers to work in partnership with transparent communication channels which enable sharing information and joint decision making between healthcare practitioners, the child when applicable, and the family, the premise being what best meets the child's needs. In healthcare practice, working in partnership with the family, who generally know the child better than others, has a number of strengths in supporting parents in general and also at times of crisis. For newly emerging parents with limited experience of caring for a child this partnership is important. Family-centred care has the potential to facilitate and enable parents to take charge of meeting their child's holistic needs whether in receipt of universal or more targeted interventions.

Family-centred care would appear to have some usefulness in the delivery of healthcare despite the refocusing of child social welfare policies to address the rights of children. Greater emphasis is now placed on the role and responsibilities of parents to care for their children, placing the child's interests and needs at the heart of decision making. It is perhaps timely to focus attention of the defining concepts of family-centred care to ensure that the needs of children, their parents and the wider family are identified, addressed and proportionally represented.

Reflective activity

Reflecting on the legislative and policy direction, compare and contrast the roles and responsibilities of parents and healthcare practitioners towards children in their care.

DEFINING FAMILY-CENTRED CARE TODAY

Shields remains one of the most prolific writers on family-centred care and its application in healthcare practice. She along with colleagues defined family-centred care as

> a way of caring for children and their families within health services which ensures that care is planned around the whole family, not just the individual child/person and in which all the family members are recognised as care recipients. (Shields et al. 2006: 1318)

This definition identifies the need to plan care around the needs of the family in which the child is situated. However, there are a number of limitations which need to be considered. There is an emphasis on all family members being viewed as recipients of care yet there is little within this definition to emphasise the dynamic movement, interaction and communication between all relevant parties. Further, there is little to emphasis the centrality of the child. The need to re-focus family-centred care through explicitly identifying the child within the context of care delivery perhaps relates significantly to what Franck and Callery (2004) suggest is the need to 're-think' family-centred care approaches in children's healthcare. Inclusion of the 'child' within a definition of family-centred care would do much to remind parents and practitioners of the need to keep the child at the centre of all decision making. Article 3 of the Convention on the Rights of the Child states:

> In all actions concerning children, whether undertaken by public or private social welfare institutions, courts of law, administrative authorities or legislative bodies, the best interests of the child shall be a primary consideration. (United Nations 1989: Article 3)

Further, Article 12 of the Convention states:

> Parties shall assure to the child who is capable of forming his or her own views the right to express those views freely in all matters affecting the child, the views of the child being given due weight in accordance with the age and maturity of the child. (United Nations 1989: Article 12)

Kelly et al. (2012) identified unexplored tensions between child-centred and family-centred models of care in children's healthcare settings. The authors suggest that such tensions need to be addressed in order to gain from models of care that best serve the child within the family.

With this point in mind, an alternative to Shield et al.'s (2006) definition is taken from the Institute of Patient and Family-Centred Care (IPFCC), which states that

> Patient and family-centered care is an approach to the planning, delivery, and evaluation of healthcare that is grounded in mutually beneficial partnerships among healthcare providers, patients, and families. It redefines the relationships in healthcare. (IPFCC 2012)

This definition emphasises not only the family but also the individual, identified as the patient, who is living within the context of the family. A further significant element is the noting of a third party, namely healthcare providers. A further strength of this second definition is the identification and inclusion of activities which, in order to have a successful outcome, require interaction between all parties. Such interaction creates a dynamism which is perhaps lacking in Shield et al.'s definition. A limitation of adopting and applying this definition is the inclusion of the term 'patient'. This point is important to consider; however, it is possible to replace 'patient' with 'child', therefore maintaining the centrality of the child within the context of the family.

There are a number of added elements within the definition offered by the IPFCC. The first is that the Institute has updated the population it endeavours to accommodate through changing its focus from family-centred to incorporate both the needs of the patient (child) and the family.

The IPFCC's definition offers a means of framing practice, not only in healthcare but also within other universal services. The application of child and family-centred care by practitioners who work in some capacity with children and their families provides an ideal framework for early interventions to support parents with a spectrum of needs to care for their child in a safe and developmentally sensitive manner. Child and family-centred care (CFCC) when applied in practice can support the best interests of the child.

One of the tensions of using family-centred care has been the inability of some nurses to accept parents as contributors in their child's care. The next section reviews the literature regarding the application of family-centred care in healthcare from the perspectives of healthcare practitioners and parents.

Reflective activity

Reflecting on your present area of clinical practice, would you consider the IPFCC's definition to fit with how practitioners frame their interaction with patients and family?

LITERATURE REVIEW OF FAMILY-CENTRED CARE WITHIN HEALTHCARE

Family-centred care is now accepted almost universally as the ideal model on which to base paediatric care, particularly in recent years where there has been an increase in the number of children living at home with chronic, long-term conditions. However, it is interesting to examine the research base providing the evidence to support this approach to child care. A wide range of research studies have been conducted which have investigated the perceptions of parents, families, children and health professionals towards family-centred care. Moore et al. (2009) conclude that

> a growing body of literature suggests that the use of interpersonal FCC [family-centred care] strategies (e.g. respect for the family's perspective) is associated with higher levels of parental satisfaction with care, improved parental well-being and reduced parental stress ... There is less evidence of the impact of FCC strategies on child outcomes. However, available studies indicate that children exhibit more developmental gains and better psychological adjustment as a result of interpersonal FCC strategies. (2009: 455)

A systematic review conducted by Shields et al. (2006) assessed the effects of family-centred care for hospitalised children, comparing standard or professionally-centred models of care on child, family and health service outcomes. The researchers failed to locate any studies that matched the inclusion criteria. The authors concluded that whilst there was a large body of literature available on the subject of family-centred care, much of this was anecdotal and descriptive, lacking in scientific rigor. A later review concluded that

> No empirical evidence exists to say FCC works or that it makes a difference to family and child healthcare outcomes. (Foster et al. 2010: 1185)

However, this is perhaps due to the challenges inherent in trying to establish direct cause-and-effect relationships in a concept as complex as family-centred care. It is difficult to design an empirical study that controls all the variables within a situation so that a direct relationship between improved health outcomes and a family-centred approach to care can be established, although a small number of studies have attempted to do so.

Improved child outcomes and family-centred care

A systematic review by Kuhlthau et al. (2011) of evidence for family-centred care for children with special healthcare needs discusses four randomised control trials, three of which demonstrated some improved health outcomes for children where a family-centred approach had been adopted. These include better personal adjustments scores (Stein and Jessop 1991), better peak flow recordings for children with asthma (Guendelman et al. 2002) and a decline in internalising symptoms amongst children with a traumatic brain injury (Wade et al. 2006). A fourth randomised trial discussed by Kuhlthau et al. of an intervention for children with attention deficit hyperactivity disorder (ADHD) demonstrated no improvement in behavioural symptoms (Wolraich et al. 2005). Kuhlthau et al. also discuss other non-randomised trials which tried to establish a link between a family-centred approach and improved child outcomes. A number of these have investigated missed school days with mixed results. Palfrey et al. (2004) did not find any differences when using a pre- and post- intervention study, whilst Farmer et al. (2005) in a similar study did find a reduction in missed school days. In another study of children with asthma, Mangione-Smith et al. (2005) showed that children who participated in a collaborative approach to care exhibited better general health-related and asthma-specific quality of life scores compared to a control group.

Moore et al. (2009) undertook an exploratory study to investigate the effect of family-centred care on health-related quality of life (HRQL) outcomes in children attending paediatric neurosciences clinics at a hospital in Canada. These children had a variety of health problems, including brain tumours, traumatic brain injury, hydrocephalus, neuromuscular disease, epilepsy and myelomeningocele. Using a variety of validated data collection tools, Moore et al. demonstrated that the level of family-centred care provided positively influenced psycho-social aspects of health-related quality of life indicators, and to a lesser degree physical indicators. However, the authors recognise that parental rather than the child's reports of HRQL are measured and that this is a limitation of the study. Kuo et al. (2011) examined the link between family-centred care and specific healthcare service outcomes for children with special healthcare needs using data from the 2005–2006 National Survey of Children with Special Healthcare Needs in the United States. The authors found that a family-centred approach to care decreases family burden and results in more efficient use of healthcare services by the child and family. In particular family-centred care was associated with positive financial factors such as less financial burden in terms of having to stop work to care for the child, out of pocket expenses, care co-ordination and direct care provision. Families also reported more stable health needs, fewer attendances at emergency departments and a reduction in behavioural problems. The authors suggest that these positive benefits are a result of improved knowledge and skills of the child's care providers within the family-centred philosophy.

The literature linking improved child outcomes to family-centred care may be as yet under developed. More evidence has been generated regarding parental perceptions of family-centred care and satisfaction with services adopting this approach to care provision.

Parental perceptions

The measure of processes of care (MPOC) is a quantitative survey tool originally developed by King et al. (1995, 1996) as a means of measuring parental perceptions of family-centred care provision. This tool has subsequently been used in many studies, translated into 5 different languages and used in 23 countries. The original survey consisted of 56 items designed to measure parents' views of family-centred behaviours displayed by health professionals. A shorter 20-item survey (MPOC-20) was subsequently developed and also a 27-item version (MPOC-SP) designed to measure service providers' perceptions (Dickens et al. 2011). The tool has been established worldwide as the most reliable indicator of family-centredness.

In an Australian study, Dickens et al. (2011) used the MPOC-20 and MPOC-SP to investigate perceptions of family-centred care within the paediatric rehabilitation services of one urban children's teaching hospital. Overall parents viewed the provision of family-centred care positively, particularly in relation to the provision of respectful and supportive care, although providing general information was seen as an area requiring improvement. Dickens et al. say that this supports the findings of two earlier studies within the Australian context (Dyke et al. 2006; Raghavendra et al. 2007). It also supports the findings of Wilkins et al. (2010) in another Australian study. Interestingly, providing general information was rated the lowest in the service providers' version of the survey. The authors suggest that a lack of time and resources may be to blame, but the findings do highlight that effective communication is an issue – a theme repeated in other studies investigating family-centred care provision.

In a literature review of 30 research studies investigating the development of family-centred care, Harrison (2010) found a common theme: parents wanted to be involved in caring for their child and recognised the need to develop a positive relationship with health professionals to achieve this outcome. However, this was problematic in many situations where nursing staff were perceived as having control of that relationship. Developing a collaborative approach to the child's care was challenging when the nurses had the power to control participation in providing care and interaction between the parent and child. This reflects the earlier findings of Corlett and Twycross (2006), who in their literature review discovered that equal partnerships often do not exist between parents and health professionals (Dearmun 1992), with parents often feeling disempowered and deskilled (Darbyshire 1994). Nurses have the power to control the communication process in order to manipulate parents into engaging in what they regard as appropriate behaviour (Callery and Smith 1991; Kawik 1996; Newton 2000), controlling the parents contribution to caring for their child (Blower and Morgan 2000). In effect, nursing staff act as gatekeepers to the child (Tomlinson et al. 2002), choosing whether or not to negotiate with the parents and family (Kirk 2001) and allow them to be partners in caring for their child.

This seems to suggest that nursing staff are rather Machiavellian in their dealings with parents, exerting their professional power and knowledge to exclude parents from interacting with and caring for their child. However, research has demonstrated that health professionals are often oblivious to the influence they have over the communication and negotiation process and are unaware of the way in which they control interaction (Brown and Ritchie 1990; Simons 2002). This is rather different from the findings of Darbyshire (1994), who in his seminal study comments that nurses actually have very clear expectations of parents; the problem is that they do not articulate these to parents who are then left to work out the ground rules for themselves in an ad hoc way, a finding reiterated by other researchers (Coyne 1995; Kawik 1996).

Over time parents become more assertive and adept at negotiating with health professionals, therefore shifting the power balance (Neill 1996; Kirk 2001). There is a recurring theme throughout all of these research studies suggesting that, if not an overt power struggle between health professionals and families, there is at least a distinct lack of clear unambiguous communication with regard to roles and expectations. Full participation and engagement of the family, a concept at the heart of genuine family-centred care, seems problematic in much of the research undertaken to date.

Health professional perspectives

Studies conducted during the 1970s to the 1990s concluded that a positive attitude towards parental participation in care by health professionals was more evident in staff who were highly educated, married, parents and occupying a senior position within the healthcare organisation (Corlett and Twycross 2006). Negative attitudes resulted from a fear of losing professional control and a lack of interpersonal and communication skills. Research conducted by Coyne (2007) indicates that whilst nurses accept the need for parents to be involved in caring for their child, they have to comply with ward norms and not disrupt the daily routine. Nurses have role expectations of parents in terms of being helpful, co-operative and undemanding. Nurses find parents who do not comply with these norms extremely disruptive and stressful to deal with, labelling them as 'problem parents' or 'nightmare families'. Parents appear to only be tolerated by the nurses as a means of getting through the workload, rather than because their involvement benefits the child and family. They conclude that

> parent participation as it is practised is clearly about administrative efficiency, not consumer empowerment (Coyne 2007: 3157)

and suggest that nurses need to develop coping, rather than communication skills. Coyne's findings reiterate the issues of power and control inherent within many studies investigating family-centred care. Unlike some earlier studies suggesting that nurses are unaware of the way in which they can manipulate and control situations, Coyne's study suggests that nurses overtly apply strategies aimed at forcing parents into complying with their professional expectations.

In a review of studies from both developed and developing countries, Foster et al. (2010) found that in many of the studies examined, a shared role in caring for a sick child resulted from a lack of adequate resources rather than negotiation or collaboration on the part of health professionals. Parents and family members often have to become involved in care, regardless of their personal wishes. It would seem that family-centred care is in danger of being highjacked as a means of maintaining service provision, rather than promoting the best interests of the child and family.

Reflective activity

What knowledge and skills do you consider practitioners require to facilitate and deliver family-centred care in your clinical area?

A SYNTHESIS OF THE EVIDENCE

The UNCRC (United Nations 1989) stated that every child has the right to experience family life. Legislation throughout the United Kingdom identified the roles and responsibilities of parents towards meeting their children's needs. It therefore appears reasonable to consider that parents have a right to receive information relating to their child as well as contributing to decisions regarding their care. Parents also need to be guided to ensure that their child is safe from significant harm. This is best achieved in an environment that facilitates learning, openness and trust.

All of these elements enable parents to fulfil their parenting role through the delivery of their parental responsibilities. However, there appears to be an incongruent approach to supporting parents because of the abstract separation of children from their parents through child-centric policies. While it is crucial to uphold a child-centred approach in all social welfare policies impacting on children, there is also a need to support families to ensure that their rights are respected, thereby supporting their ability to address the needs of their children.

The adoption of a child- and family-centred care framework identifies the child, parents and practitioners as contributing to meeting the needs of the child within the family context. There are no other frameworks available which ensure that parents are supported to meet their parenting responsibilities. Therefore adopting a framework of this nature appears to be a pertinent way forward as a universal intervention and if necessary can provide a platform for the provision of more targeted interventions.

While there is clearly a need for further research to conclusively determine outcomes, there appears to be sufficient evidence supporting the continued adoption of the family-centred approach to child care. Four inter-related emerging themes that need to be addressed in order to practice child- and family-centred care are: the culture in which healthcare is delivered; professional communication; educational preparation of practitioners; and adequate resources to practice. These are discussed below.

EMERGING THEMES

Culture

The culture in which nursing and midwifery practitioners engage with children and their families has changed over the years. There is now evidence supporting positive changes to the culture in which children and their families are cared for. However, evidence to the contrary continues to raise concerns, as in the recent case of Hayley Fullerton who died aged 13 months in Birmingham Children's Hospital in 2011 (Paduano 2012).

The literature review identified that there are practitioners who fail to work in partnership with parents. Powerful dominance over parents by some practitioners in relation to care delivery remains evident. Such cultural beliefs, values and attitudes do not support safeguarding children. There is, however, evidence of good practice where examples of parents and family members working in partnership with practitioners works well.

When considering safeguarding children from harm the underpinning professional culture is central to bringing about the necessary changes in practices (Munro 2011). To facilitate a culture change in order to enhance positive outcomes for children and their families requires transformational leadership along with the introduction of structures and processes which empower, develop and evaluate the care delivered by practitioners (Manley 2004). Incorporating an approach or framework to guiding child-centred care within the context of the family needs to be underpinned by a culture which embraces the values of all stakeholders and not just the views of professionals.

The literature review identified that both the family and professionals have a part to play in caring for a child. However, the emphasis and control still appears to be with the health professionals, and in many cases, according to the research, there is a continuing need to respect the family and the contribution they can make. Empathic and facilitative communicative interaction between parents and practitioners can be viewed as a positive step in the prevention of child maltreatment. Equally, family-centred care could offer the first early intervention to support parents in meeting the welfare and developmental needs of their child.

Professional communication

The second emerging theme from this review is the quality of professional communication. While it has long been recognised that skilful and empathic communication is central when caring for children, families and other patient groups, the evidence relating to family-centred care suggests that the quality of communicative interaction was poor and at times ineffective. There are two specific elements underpinning effective communication which need to be addressed. The first is the delivery of all information to parents relating to their child. Such information should be delivered in a manner that enhances parental understanding and enables parents to contribute to the decision making process (Department of Health 2001). In the event of a child who is developmentally capable of making or contributing to making decisions, parents who remain responsible need sufficient information in order to support their child. This last point is supported through legislation relating to the care of children within the United Kingdom.

A further consideration regarding communication is the relational function of communication. Munro (2011) identified how interaction with parents has to change. There needs to be greater efforts by practitioners to form relationships with parents and children in order to meet the needs of the child. It is only through such relationships that transparent and honest communication can take place. The relational aspect of care requires nurses and midwives to have the ability to skilfully apply the art and science of communication to maximise effective working relationships. This is crucial to safeguarding the needs of children within the family context.

Education

The third emerging theme is the inclusion of robust educational programmes addressing the culture in which care delivery is managed as well as addressing the relational aspects of care. As healthcare in general, and child and family care in particular, moves towards more inclusive ways of working with individuals and families, greater effort is needed to enable practitioners to develop and apply the necessary knowledge, understanding and skills which will embrace inclusive practices.

Further, the need for education about family-centred care has been identified in this review. Perhaps this is as much about fostering appropriate values and attitudes through undergraduate education and then through continuing professional development, rather than simply identifying the underpinning principles of this approach to child care. In this way a positive culture can be fostered in which practitioners work as partners in providing child-centric care. Education also needs to embrace an inter-professional approach in which these values and attitudes are shared across traditional role boundaries via shared learning and continuing professional development opportunities.

Appropriate resourcing

A final emerging theme relates to appropriate resourcing of healthcare services. It is apparent in much of the research that the successful implementation of a genuinely family-centred approach to care requires adequate resourcing, particularly in terms of sufficient numbers of appropriately training staff. Engaging in positive communication and fostering a collaborative approach to care with families requires time, which is often limited due to chronic staff shortages and the resulting pressure on daily tasks. When taking this into consideration, it is understandable that staff such as those in Coyne's (2007) study need parents to be compliant. Staff then become frustrated when parents do not comply with ward expectations. It is important to recognise that adopting a family-centred philosophy of care provision can be both expensive and resource intensive, and there must be support at senior management level in order for it to be successful. However, it also has to be recognised that precious resources are often unwittingly squandered as a result of the way in which staff carry out their duties and the way in which the ward is organised. The *Releasing Time to Care: The Productive Ward* initiative (NHS Institute for Innovation and Improvement 2007; NHS Scotland 2008) has demonstrated how much time is wasted by staff on activities such as searching for equipment, borrowing supplies and unnecessary walking around the ward area, due to the way the ward is organised. With some thought and re-organisation better use of staff time will allow for direct patient care and interaction. There is obviously a need to recognise that a family-centred approach to care requires time to communicate and build relationships with families; the answer may be to not only campaign for more staff but also to rethink the way in which the ward environment is organised, ensuring efficiency in all areas. Another dimension to this, specific to a family-centred approach, is to think about how the ward environment affects the delivery of family-centred care. In a qualitative study Beck et al. (2009) discovered that the physical environment affected the delivery of family-centred care. Small rooms suitable for one child and family members, equipped with a bed for the parent, were more facilitative than open multiple-bed bays as they provided private, quiet areas for staff to talk to parents and build relationships with them.

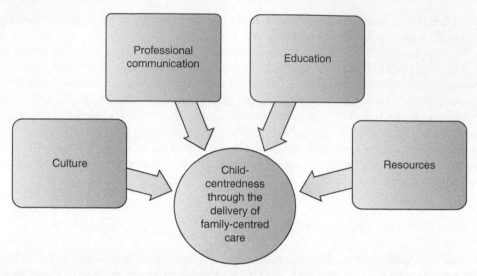

Figure 7.1 Addressing emerging themes to facilitate child-centredness through family-centred care by nursing and midwifery practitioners

Figure 7.1 presents a framework of the emerging themes identified from the literature review. Four inter-related emerging themes which appeared to support or constrain the practice of family-centred care are identified.

CASE STUDY

Patrick is three years of age and lives with his mum Sharon, dad Jim, and brother Gregor. In his short life, Patrick has experienced two episodes of bowel obstruction which required hospitalisation and surgery. Since the last episode, Patrick and his family have moved to another part of the country due to his dad's job.

After settling into their new home the family health visitor arranged to visit after receiving notification of Patrick and his family's registration with their new general practitioner. Sharon was pleased to meet their new health visitor but was anxious throughout the visit. She broke down in tears when telling the health visitor about Patrick's episodes of illness. Sharon stated that when Patrick was admitted to hospital both she and Jim were not encouraged to stay with him. Patrick was often separated from Sharon and Jim for long periods. They were not kept informed of his condition but had to ask for updates on his progress. One time Patrick's condition deteriorated when they were visiting him and the nurses directed them to leave and phone back later. They were not allowed to carry out any of Patrick's care during his hospital stays. Sharon told the health visitor that both she and Patrick's dad lost confidence in caring for Patrick and both became very anxious, which impacted on their health. They found these experiences very traumatic, causing them to shelter Patrick from new experiences for fear of something happening to him. Patrick was very clingy with his mum and reluctant to interact with others.

Just after Sharon's meeting with the health visitor, Patrick received an appointment to visit the paediatric clinic in a new hospital for a check-up. After reviewing Patrick's condition, the new surgeon advised Sharon and Jim that Patrick would do better with a colostomy because of adhesions which, more than likely, would lead to further episodes of obstruction. Sharon and Jim were devastated but realised that the surgeon was doing what was right for Patrick. Both parents were extremely anxious for Patrick and his imminent hospitalisation. Sharon contacted the health visitor and informed her of Patrick's pending admission. The health visitor reassured Sharon that their experiences would be different. The health visitor contacted the paediatric ward to liaise with nursing staff.

Child and family-centred care approach

Patrick was admitted to the paediatric ward the day before his operation. On entering the ward, the family were surprised to see a brightly coloured and open reception area which appeared busy with children, parents and staff. Sharon noted large posters on the wall stating the philosophy of how children and their families were cared for. A particular poster caught Sharon's attention because it was headed by the term 'family-centred care' in large bold red print. Both Sharon and Jim, though remaining anxious, were happy to be surrounded by such a vibrant, happy and colourful environment. They felt more at ease after reading the posters on the wall.

The family were greeted by a nurse who introduced herself as Jane and shook the hands of both parents. Jane informed Sharon and Jim she would be caring for Patrick and his family throughout Patrick's stay in hospital. Jane appeared friendly and approachable, respecting and acknowledging Sharon and Jim's obvious anxiety. The family were shown around the brightly coloured ward before being shown into a side room with a small bed for Patrick and a bed for a member of his family. Jane informed the family that they were very family friendly and worked in partnership with parents, other family members, as well as other practitioners such as physiotherapists, play specialists and community staff. Sharon and Jim were very pleased to hear this. Jane said that the family health visitor had been in touch with the ward and would be coming up to visit the family. They were advised about meals and if they preferred to prepare meals for themselves and their children there was a kitchen close by.

Jane completed Patrick's care-plan in partnership with Sharon who had selected to remain with Patrick. Sharon explained to Jane about her experiences and anxieties resulting from Patrick's earlier admissions. Jane was very reassuring, explaining that the staff in this ward worked differently, preferring to work in partnership with parents. The surgeon who was to operate on Patrick spent time with Sharon,

(Continued)

(Continued)

Jim and Patrick, discussing the operation and explaining in detail what to expect before and after surgery. Patrick was later examined in preparation for his operation by an anaesthetist who communicated with Sharon, listening to her account of Patrick's general health and previous surgeries. Later, the specialist stoma nurse and Jane involved Sharon and Jim in the discussion about where the colostomy should be located on Patrick's abdomen. This had previously also been discussed with the surgeon.

Sharon and Jim were encouraged to participate in Patrick's pre- and post-operative care, which included comforting Patrick before and after surgery. They contributed to decisions relating to Patrick's need for pain relief, fluids and food, activity, comfort and play. Jane and the stoma specialist worked in partnership with Sharon and Jim to help build their confidence in managing Patrick's stoma. This was an intensive activity as neither parent had had any prior experience of stoma care. They responded positively to joining a parent stoma support group before leaving hospital.

Prior to discharge, Patrick and his parents met with their health visitor, Jane and the stoma specialist to identify any potential difficulties. Sharon and Jim were provided with contact information should they need support, an outpatients appointment and leaflets advising about Patrick's health, development and stoma care.

Before leaving the paediatric ward Sharon and Jim were asked to complete an evaluation questionnaire regarding their stay. They were advised that this information would be used to assess the quality of care provided to both children and their families in that ward.

CONCLUSION

This chapter has addressed the application of family-centred care in the healthcare setting. Other approaches offering the same or similar guidance for healthcare practitioners and families could not be identified. In light of recent legislation, which makes explicit the roles and responsibilities of parents towards their children, as well as contemporary child care policies, it is perhaps timely to reconsider the properties and definition of family-centredness. Supporting parents to fulfil their roles and responsibilities to meet their child's holistic needs is a necessary part of healthcare practitioners' work. Redefining family-centred care to child and family centred care therefore needs to be considered as a way forward. Evolving family-centred care towards child and family approaches maintains the child at the centre of care while acknowledging the role and therefore needs of parents.

From the evidence presented in this chapter, more research to identify the effectiveness of the family-centred approach to care for children through a partnership of parents and practitioners is warranted. A review of the literature identified the need to address the limitations of culture, professional communication, education of nurses and midwives, as well as the provision of adequate resources to engage with children and their parents to promote positive outcomes for all stakeholders.

FURTHER READING

Department for Education (1989) *The Children Act*. London: HMSO.
Northern Ireland Assembly (1995) *The Children (Northern Ireland) Order*. Stormont: Northern Ireland Assembly.
Scottish Executive (1995) *The Children (Scotland) Act*. Edinburgh: Scottish Executive.

REFERENCES

Allen, G. (2011) *Early Intervention: The Next Steps. An Independent Report to Her Majesty's Government*. London: Cabinet Office.
Beck, S., Weis, J., Greisen, G., Anderson, M. and Zoffmann, V. (2009) Room for family-centered care – a qualitative evaluation of a neonatal intensive care unit remodeling project. *Journal of Neonatal Nursing* 15: 88–99.
Blower, K. and Morgan, E. (2000) Great expectations? Parental participation in care. *Journal of Child Healthcare* 4(2): 60–65.
Bowlby, J. (1944a) Forty-four juvenile thieves: Their characters and home life. *International Journal of Psycho-analysis* 25: 19–53.
Bowlby, J. (1944b) Forty-four juvenile thieves: Their characters and home life (ii). *International Journal of Psycho-analysis* 25: 107–127.
Brandon, M., Sidebotham, P., Ellis, C., Bailey, S. and Belderson, P. (2011) *Child and Family Practitioners' Understanding of Child Development: Lessons Learnt from a Small Sample of Serious Case Reviews*. London: Department of Education.
Britto, P. and Ulkuer, N. (2012) Child development in developing countries: Child rights and policy implications. *Child Development* 83(1): 92–103.
Brown, J. and Ritchie, J. (1990) Nurses' perceptions of parent and nurse roles in caring for hospitalized children. *Child Healthcare* 19(1): 28–36.
Callery, P. and Smith, L. (1991) A study of role negotiation between nurses and the parents of hospitalized children. *Journal of Advanced Nursing* 16: 772–781.
Casey, A. (1993) Development and use of the partnership model of nursing care. In E. Glasper and A. Tucker (eds), *Advances in Child Health Nursing*. Oxford: Scutari. pp. 183–193.
Cawson, P. (2002) *Child Maltreatment in the Family: The Experience of a National Sample of Young People*. London: NSPCC.
Corlett, J. and Twycross, A. (2006) Negotiation of parental roles within family-centred care: A review of the research. *Journal of Clinical Nursing* 15(10): 1308–1316.
Coyne, I. (1995) Partnership in care: Parents' views of participation in their hospitalized child's care. *Journal of Clinical Nursing* 4: 71–79.
Coyne, I. (2007) Disruption of parent participation: Nurses' strategies to manage parents on children's wards. *Journal of Clinical Nursing* 17: 3150–3158.

Darbyshire, P. (1994) *Living with a Sick Child in Hospital: The Experiences of Parents and Nurses*. London: Chapman and Hall.

Dearmun, A. (1992) Perceptions of parental participation. *Paediatric Nursing* 4(7): 6–9.

Department for Education and Skills (2003) *Every Child Matters*. London: The Stationery Office.

Department of Health (2001) *The Bristol Royal Infirmary Inquiry: The Kennedy Report*. London: The Stationery Office.

Dickens, K., Matthews, L. and Thompson, J. (2011) Parent and service providers' perceptions regarding the delivery of family-centred paediatric rehabilitation services in a children's hospital. *Child: Care, Health and Development* 37: 64–73.

Dyke, P., Buttigieg, P., Blackmore, A. and Ghose, A. (2006) Use of the measure of process of care for families (MPOC-56) and service providers (MPOC-SP) to evaluate family-centred services in a paediatric disability setting. *Child: Care, Health and Development* 32: 167–176.

Farmer, J., Clark, M. and Sherman, A. (2005) Comprehensive primary care for children with special healthcare needs in rural areas. *Pediatrics* 116: 649–656.

Foster, M., Whitehead, L. and Maybee, P. (2010) Parents' and health professionals' perceptions of family centred care for children in hospital, in developed and developing countries: A review of the literature. *International Journal of Nursing Studies* 47: 1184–1193.

Franck, L. and Callery, P. (2004) Re-thinking family-centred care across the continuum of children's healthcare. *Child: Care, Health and Development* 30(3): 265–277.

Glaser, D. (2011) How to deal with emotional abuse and neglect: Further development of a conceptual framework (FRAMEA). *Child Abuse and Neglect* 35: 866–875.

Guendelman, S., Meade, K., Benson, M., Chen, Y. and Samuels, S. (2002) Improving asthma outcomes and self-management behaviours of inner-city children. *Archives of Pediatric and Adolescent Medicine* 156: 115–120.

Guralnick, M. (2009) Family influences on early development: Integrating the science of normative development, risk and disability, and intervention. In K. McCartney and D. Phillips (ed.), *Blackwell Handbook of Early Childhood Development*. Oxford: Blackwell. pp. 44–61.

Hall, C., Parton, N., Peckover, S. and White, S. (2010) Child-centric information and communication technology (ICT) and the fragmentation of child welfare practice in England. *Journal of Social Policy* 39: 393–413.

Harrison, T. (2010) Family-centered pediatric nursing care: State of the science. *Journal of Pediatric Nursing* 25: 335–343.

Institute for Patient- and Family-Centred Care (IPFCC) (2012) Institute for Patient- and Family-Centred Care website. Available at: www.ipfcc.org/services/index.html (accessed 02 February 2012). Bethesda, MD: IPFCC.

Jolley, J. and Shields, L. (2009) The evolution of family-centred care. *Journal of Pediatric Nursing* 242: 164–170.

Kawik, L. (1996) Nurses' and parents' perceptions of participation and partnership in caring for a hospitalized child. *British Journal of Nursing* 5(7): 430–434.

Kelly, M., Jones, S., Wilson, V. and Lewis, P. (2012) How children's rights are constructed in family-centred care: A review of the literature. *Journal of Child Healthcare* 16: 190–205.

King, S., Rosenbaum, P. and King, G. (1995) *The Measure of Processes of Care (MPOC): A Means to Assess Family-centred Behaviours of Healthcare Providers*. Hamilton: CanChild Centre for Childhood Disability Research, McMaster University.

King, S., Rosenbaum, P. and King, G. (1996) Parents' perceptions of caregiving development and validation of a measure of processes. *Development Medicine and Child Neurology* 38: 757–772.

Kirk, S. (2001) Negotiating lay and professional roles in the care of children with complex healthcare needs. *Journal of Advanced Nursing* 34(5): 593–560.

Kuhlthau, K., Bloom, S., Van Cleave, J., Knapp, A., Romm, D., Klatka, K., Homer, C., Newacheck, P. and Perrin, J. (2011) Evidence of family-centred care for children with special healthcare needs: A systematic review. *Academic Pediatrics* 11: 136–143.

Kuo, D., Bird, T. and Tilford, J. (2011) Associations of family-centered care with healthcare outcomes for children with special healthcare needs. *Maternal Child Health* 15: 794–805.

Mangione-Smith, R., Schonlau, M., Chan, K., Keesey, J., Rosen, M., Louis, T. and Keeler, E. (2005) Measuring the effectiveness of a collaborative for quality improvement in pediatric asthma care: Does implementing the chronic care model improve processes and outcomes of care? *Ambulatory Pediatrics* 5: 75–82.

Manley, K. (2004) *Transformational Culture: A Culture of Effectiveness*. In K. McCormack, K. Manley and R. Garbett (ed.), *Practice Development in Nursing*. Oxford: Blackwell. pp. 51–82.

Ministry of Health (1959) *The Welfare of Children in Hospital: Platt Report*. London: HMSO.

Moore, M., Mah, J. and Trute, B. (2009) Family-centred care and health-related quality of life of patients in paediatric neurosciences. *Child: Care Health and Development* 35: 454–461.

Munro, E. (2011) *The Munro Review of Child Protection: Final Report: A Child-centred System*. London: Department of Education.

Neill, S. (1996) Parent participation 2: Findings and their implications for practice. *British Journal of Nursing* 5(2): 110–117.

Newton, M. (2000) Family-centred care: Current realities in parent participation. *Pediatric Nursing* 26(2): 164–168.

NHS Institute for Innovation and Improvement (2007) *The Productive Ward: Releasing Time to Care*. London: NHS Institute for Innovation and Improvement.

NHS Scotland (2008) *Releasing Time to Care: The Productive Ward*. Edinburgh: NHS Scotland.

Northern Ireland Assembly (2006) *Our Children and Young People – Our Shared Responsibility: The Reform Implementation Process in Child Protection Services in Northern Ireland*. Belfast: Department of Health, Social Services and Public Safety.

Paduano, M. (2012) Hayley Fullerton: 'Hospital failings' ahead of death. 10 December 2012. Available at: www.bbc.co.uk/news/uk-england-birmingham-20323760 (accessed October 2013).

Palfrey, J., Solis, L. and Davidson, E. (2004) The pediatric alliance for coordinated care: Evaluation of a medical home model. *Pediatrics* 113: 1507–1516.

Raghavendra, P., Murchland, S., Bently, M., Wake-Dyster, W. and Lyons, T. (2007) Parents' and service providers' perceptions of family-centred practice in a community-based, paediatric disability service in Australia. *Child: Care, Health and Development* 33: 586–592.

Scottish Executive (2005) *Getting it Right for Every Child: Proposals for Action*. Edinburgh: Scottish Executive.

Shields, L. (2010) Questioning family-centred care. *Journal of Clinical Nursing* 19: 2629–2638.

Shields, L., Pratt, J. and Hunter, J. (2006) Family-centred care: A review of qualitative studies. *Journal of Clinical Nursing* 15: 1317–1323.

Simons, J. (2002) Parents' support and satisfaction with their child's postoperative care. *British Journal of Nursing* 11(22): 1442–1449.

Stein, R. and Jessop, D. (1991) Long-term mental health effects of a pediatric home care program. *Pediatrics* 88: 490–496.

Sutherland, E. (2001) Care of the child within the family. In A. Sutherland (ed.), *Children's Rights in Scotland*, 2nd edn. Edinburgh: Green. pp. 91–103.

Tomlinson, P., Thomlinson, E., Pedine-McAlpine, C. and Kirschbaum, M. (2002) Clinical innovation for promoting family care in paediatric intensive care: Demonstration, role modeling and reflective practice. *Journal of Advanced Nursing* 38: 161–170.

United Nations (1989) *United Nations Convention on the Rights of the Child*. Geneva: United Nations.

Wade, S., Michaud, L. and Brown, T. (2006) Putting the pieces together: Preliminary efficacy of a family problem-solving intervention for children with traumatic brain injury. *Journal of Head Trauma Rehabilitation* 21: 57–67.

Welsh Assembly Government (2004) *Children and Young People: From Rights to Action*. Cardiff: Welsh Assembly Government.

Wilkins, A., Leonard, H., Jacoby, P., MacKinnon, E., Clohessy, P., Forouhgi, S. and Slack-Smith, L. (2010) Evaluation of the processes of family-centred care for young children with intellectual disability in Western Australia. *Child: Care, Health and Development* 36: 709–718.

Wolraich, M., Bickman, L. and Lambert, E. (2005) Intervening to improve communication between parents, teachers, and primary care providers of children with ADHD or at high risk of ADHD. *Journal of Attention Disorders* 9: 354–368.

8

ENGAGING WITH CHILDREN, YOUNG PEOPLE AND THEIR FAMILIES

SANDRA RODWELL AND GILL WATSON

CHAPTER SUMMARY

Communication is the cornerstone to engaging with, assessing and understanding the needs of children, young people and their families. Communication is defined as the exchange of thoughts, information or messages (Levetown 2008) using a number of communicative processes that are verbal, for example talking, or non-verbal, such as writing, drawing and possibly observing. Generally, communication is a two-way process between two individuals or groups of people. However, one exception to this is when one person is observing another without the observed being aware. This one-sided communication is common when observing a child's behaviour within a specific environment, which may include interacting with parents or other children. Observing patterns of child behaviour can communicate the level of vulnerability (secure or insecure) the child is experiencing.

Engaging with children and their families is central to safe and effective practice in safeguarding and protecting children. In line with current policies (*Every Child Matters*, Department of Education and Skills 2003; *Getting it Right for Every*

Child, Scottish Executive 2005; *Children and Young People: Rights to Action*, Welsh Assembly Government 2004; and *Our Children and Young People, Our Shared Responsibility: The Reform Implementation Process in Child Protection Services in Northern Ireland*, Northern Ireland Assembly 2006), the process of engagement should include meaningful interaction with children and young people. Children and young people need information about any issues that may be impacting on their lives in a format they can understand. At the same time they need to have the opportunity to express their feelings and talk about their experiences so that these are taken into account when decisions are being made that affect them. Children may also need information about any support that is available to them. To engage requires communication, and to communicate with a child or young person requires a relationship of trust and respect. A relationship which is underpinned by these qualities is more likely to allow the child's views to be heard and considered. Developing such a relationship requires particular skills as children and young people have different levels of ability to participate in conversations. Much is dependent upon a wide variety of factors, including their developmental stage, vocabulary and reasoning ability, culture, social norms and context. The level of awareness of individual practitioners as to the appropriate adjustments they may have to make to their approach in response to these factors is an essential component of a successful interaction.

This chapter identifies the conventions, legislation and policies underpinning the reasons for engaging with children and young people. The principles and practice of effective communication, the barriers to effective communication and the qualities and skills required when engaging in both everyday conversations and those involving sensitive issues surrounding child safeguarding and protection will be discussed.

It is important to consider communication not only with children and young people but also with their parents or carers. Adults also have varying needs regarding communication which practitioners should assess and respond to appropriately. Using effective communication models can enhance the efficacy of other assessment processes, such as those guided by the My World Triangle (Department of Health 2000), an assessment framework discussed previously in Chapter 6. This aids the initiation of communication between agency involvement to ensure that the initial needs of all are met.

It is not of the intention of this chapter to provide advice regarding counselling or therapeutic treatment of a child or young person who has been subjected to any form of abuse or neglect. Neither does this chapter provide a comprehensive guide on how to use specific tools, for example Makaton, sign language or talking mats. This chapter raises awareness about the importance of what is essentially the most commonly used tool in practice and its impact on effective and efficient care.

Within this chapter the term 'child' or 'children' should be taken to include infants, children or young people between the ages of 0–18 years old as set out by Article 1 of the United Nations Convention on the Rights of the Child (United Nations 1989). These terms are used interchangeably.

AIMS OF THIS CHAPTER

This chapter has two aims. The first aim is raise awareness of the significance communication plays in interaction between children, parents and practitioners, regardless of the focus for communicating. The second aim is to discuss the principles and styles of communicative interactions that can be used to address the safeguarding and protective needs of children and young people.

Learning outcomes

After reading this chapter and following a period of reflection the reader will be able to:

- Define and discuss the meaning of communication and the impact communication can have on child and family welfare outcomes.
- Identify the key components of effective engagement and communication with children, young people and their parents.
- Critically review the place of communication when safeguarding and protecting children and young people.
- Develop self-awareness of your own communicative practice when interacting with children, young people and their families.

Key words

enabling; engagement; listening; therapeutic relationship; understanding; verbal and non-verbal communication

As discussed previously in Chapter 1, the rights-based agenda arose out of the European Convention on Human Rights (1950) and the United Nations Convention on the Rights of the Child (1989), which repositioned child welfare and the social status of children and young people within the United Kingdom. The resulting legislation and policies in Scotland (*Getting it Right for Every Child*, Scottish Executive 2005), England (*Every Child Matters*, Department of Education and Skills 2003), Wales (*Children and Young People: Rights to Action*, Welsh Assembly Government 2004) and Northern Ireland (*Our Children and Young People, Our Pledge: The Reform Implementation Process in Child Protection Services in Northern Ireland* (Northern Ireland Assembly 2006) acknowledge the rights of children and young people not only to be protected from harm in every aspect of their lives, but also the right to be heard (United Nations 1989: Article 12), freedom to express their views (1989: Article 13) and the right to information relating to themselves (1989 Article 17).

The impact of these wide-reaching legislative and political reforms has implication for all institutions and organisations at the heart of British society as well as those sitting on the periphery. Practitioners from all universal services are now required to adopt child-centred practice when engaging with children, young people and their families. Children and young people now need to be communicated with to enable their views to be heard, their experiences reported and to be given information relating to their own needs.

As cited in Cossar et al. the Children's Commissioner for England states:

> Listening to the views of children and striving to understand their experiences are both fundamental to ensuring their rights to protection, support and participation under the United Nations Convention on the Rights of the Child are fully realised. We would encourage professionals to grasp this and act on it so that children feel heard and are able to engage in the process of protection. Such understanding is also vital to the assessment which is made of their needs. (2011: 4)

This statement underlines the importance of practitioners engaging children and young people in meaningful communication exchanges. This may be particularly challenging in situations where a child or young person has a sensory or cognitive condition which requires specific tools to augment communication, for example sign language, Makaton, Braille or easy-read material. In these situations there may still be a tendency for practitioners to look to the parent or carer to mediate on their behalf, particularly in small rural or island communities where the adult may be known to the practitioner on a personal level.

Nonetheless, healthcare practitioners with access to children, whether directly or indirectly, are required to consider the individual needs of every child, regardless of their developmental stage and abilities. This situation introduces the question of assessing competency of the child and their parents. Practitioners and parents may either overestimate or underestimate a child's level of understanding. It may be that a child is fully competent in relation to one situation and not another (Beauchamp and Childress 2001). For example, a child may fully understand simple choices related to their situation but may not be able to understand the potential consequences of more complex issues. This situation may also apply to the child's parents. However, it is important that children and young people regardless of competence should feel empowered to disclose their feelings, worries and concerns in the way that they can, with adults responding appropriately in a non-judgemental manner. Corby (2006) acknowledges that whilst some boundaries and guidelines are necessary, using a child's age and understanding as a measure of competency can result in children's reports of abuse being treated with some level of doubt.

It is important to note then that when engaging with children and young people, access to other knowledge is also important and necessary. Knowledge of child development, including child behaviour and identifying secure and insecure infant–parent attachments, are just some of the other concepts practitioners need to master.

Parents too have a right to information relating to their child. This is essential if they are to fulfil their roles and responsibilities to meet the needs of their child. Their ability to do so may be dependent on their knowledge, communication skills and their own personal situation as well as cultural influences. In order to support family-centred, child-focused care, practitioners must create a communication environment which enables them to provide parents and carers with accessible information in order to ensure that parents understand their responsibilities and what they involve, and to gather appropriate information to inform the assessment process.

Understanding the purpose of all aspects of communication and its underpinning theories and models is essential in order to understand what children and young people are saying.

COMMUNICATING WITH THE CHILD OR YOUNG PERSON: PRINCIPLES AND PRACTICE

Key principles supporting effective communication

Communicating with children or young people in healthcare is most commonly associated with health or developmental examinations or when in receipt of interventions such as immunisations. There are other times, however, when conversations with children are necessary, such as when a child is known or suspected to have been exposed to significant harm. Regardless of the reason to converse with a child, it is helpful to frame and guide the interaction using a number of key principles which, according to Levetown (2008), increase the effectiveness of the communication event, including improving outcomes for the child.

The first key principle is that all communication with children needs to be child-centred and not shaped or framed by adult-style conversations. Of course, childhood transgresses a number of developmental stages across physical, cognitive, psychological and social domains from birth to the early twenties. Therefore, having an understanding of the pattern and sequence of child development abilities across all domains is necessary when preparing to engage a child in conversation.

Gaining a better understanding of how best to address the developmental needs of children is essential for practitioners in healthcare, including those delivering adult-focused services because the adult client may also be a parent. The children may or may not be at higher risk of exposure to harm (Cuthbert and Stanley 2012).

The second key principle is that a holistic approach to communication (Kolucki and Lemish 2011) must be used when dealing with children, young people and their families. Applying this in practice requires the communicative process to consider the implications of the interaction with the child along their physical, psychological, social and cognitive domains. For example, when sharing information with a child, it is necessary to identify how the child feels about the information whilst at the same time ensuring that the child feels physically and socially safe.

Engaging in communication with others in healthcare is possibly the most common activity undertaken when compared to all other procedures. Even when caring for a patient who has received an anaesthetic, the effective practitioner will touch and direct conversations towards the unconscious patient. Clearly, engaging with patients requires communicating in some form or other. The skills and practices used to communicate will vary in accordance with the context underpinning the engagement. The next section explores the common skills and how they are adapted when communicating with children and their parents.

TRANSLATING THEORY INTO PRACTICE

As discussed earlier in this chapter, developing a therapeutic relationship is central to engaging with children, young people and their parents. Such a relationship is powerful, goal directed and client-focused, based on trusting, empathic and ethical care (College of Registered Nurses in Nova Scotia 2012). The quality of the therapeutic relationship and the skills of practitioners will impact on the effectiveness of any interaction and subsequent outcomes for children, young people and their families.

Engaging and communicating with children and parents can be managed using three basic but skilled and interactive activities: listening, understanding and enabling, as addressed below. The application of each activity needs to be adapted in response to the context; for example, the location, environment and focus of the communication. Whether the practitioner is communicating with both child and parent or the child or parent on their own, the same activities and skills should remain child-centred and focused on the communication needs of the individual.

Listening

Effective listening by practitioners requires attention to the detail of the message delivered by the child through verbal or non-verbal means. Effective listening is the means of conveying trust (Stevenson et al. 2004) and the experience being relayed is both significant and important. Listening requires the practitioner to follow the story line without interrupting the flow of the message. Listening and hearing the experiences of the child has benefits for both child and practitioner. The practitioner's ability to convey through both non-verbal and verbal means and attention to the detail of the child's experiences has a significant bearing on the effectiveness of the interaction.

Non-verbal cues impacting on listening

- It is important to be aware of non-verbal cues in relation to respecting personal space and appropriate use of touch. Touching someone's arm, for example, may be either appropriate as a comforting gesture or not, depending upon the individual's preferences, culture and the situation (Stickley, 2011).

- Sitting side by side on a sofa or the floor can give the child the opportunity to move nearer or further away. They can also make or avoid eye contact, depending on what is more comfortable for them. This gives the child an element of control, particularly if they are about to disclose information of an intimate or difficult nature. Everyone sitting at the same level can be helpful in reducing feelings of intimidation. Conversations may also take place when a child is playing with toys, computer games or other activities that help them to relax. Adopting an open posture reinforces the message that the practitioner is interested in what the child has to say as well as indicating that they are not feeling threatened or worried about the conversation, thus encouraging further communication.
- Leaning towards a child is an indication that the practitioner is interested in what they are saying; however, it may also be interpreted as a threatening gesture. This may be particularly relevant when a child has been the subject of abuse.
- Making good eye contact is important as it informs the child that the practitioner is interested in what they have to say. However, it is important not to maintain eye contact for a prolonged time. A child could find prolonged eye contact uncomfortable or intimidating. At the same time it should be recognised that avoiding eye contact could lead to the child feeling that the practitioner is uncomfortable or distressed by what they are saying. This could result in the child feeling unable to continue with the conversation.

Verbal cues impacting on listening

- Asking questions is an important strategy to use as it further strengthens the impression to the child that their experiences have been heard. However, care must be taken not to interrupt a child who is describing their experiences. Therefore, any questions should be asked when there is a general pause in the conversation.

Reflective activity

Reflecting on your last conversation with a patient, can you identify the listening skills you used?

What other listening skills could you have used?

Understanding

While listening enables the experience to be heard, understanding involves using skills and activities that build meaning of the experience disclosed by the child. Understanding is also recognised as the basis of a therapeutic relationship, and empathy is central in

(Continued)

(Continued)

the understanding process (Rollnick et al. 2008). When the practitioner tries to build meaning and understanding of the child's experiences, it is important to view the child's experiences from their perspective (Stevenson et al. 2004).

Skills and activities to build meaning and understanding

- Asking questions to probe for more information is often used to build a better understanding of the reported experience or to identify if the child requires information. Questions may be directive or guiding in nature, depending on the context. Direct questions are often used to clarify significant points, while guiding questions can be used to explore further some aspects such as how the child feels about an experience (Stevenson et al. 2004).
- Paraphrasing can also be used to develop better understanding regarding an experience. Paraphrasing can be helpful when attempting to develop a clearer understanding of a situation but without having to ask further questions.
- The process of building a better understanding of a child's experience needs to convey some level of reassurance and support in the interactive process, but care is required so as not to convey unrealistic reassurances over outcomes.

Enabling

The activities of listening and building understanding provide a sound platform on which interactions between child and practitioner can support the child's future development. Enabling involves supporting and comforting a child through any interaction with a practitioner.

Skills and activities to comfort and enable

- Addressing uncertainty is required but without creating unrealistic expectations. It is necessary to examine the impact of uncertainties which a child may experience. It is not possible to remove all uncertainties; much will depend on the context of the child's experiences. However, it is possible to reduce the impact that uncertainties may have on a child's emotional well-being through the provision of pertinent and accurate information. It is important to avoid technical terms and complex sentence structures. Keep the communication simple, using everyday language. Sentences should focus on one instruction or piece of information at a time. This level of support can reduce the overwhelming response that uncertainty can cause.
- Supporting the child to explore positive aspects in their lives or to consider how they can best approach a new experience is important. Exploring with the child more positive sides to their lives can be helpful. Introducing a child to new activities may be of benefit.

Through the integration of listening, understanding and enabling skills when engaging with a child, the practitioner is more able to attend to the holistic needs of the child, as specified earlier under the second key principle.

The key principles and the skills presented above have been explored from the perspective of the child. However, when engaging with parents, with or without the child being present, the same principles and skills can be applied.

How to maximize engagement with children and their parents

- Gain attention
- Slow down
- Use short sentences
- Stress key words
- Pause

- Allow the person lots of processing time
- Avoid repeating too quickly
- Avoid jargon
- Use proper nouns instead of pronouns

FRAMEWORK SUPPORTING THE PROCESS OF ASSESSMENT AND COMMUNICATION

The advantage of using communication frameworks is that they provide a recognised structure or approach to information gathering and dissemination by multi-disciplinary and multi-agency teams, therefore minimising the potential for communication errors or omissions. Any framework used by practitioners should fit with the requirements of the local safeguarding policy and related communication pathways.

Reflective activity

Reflecting on your clinical area of practice, identify the communication pathways used to safeguard children and young people.

Assessment framework: a framework for assessing children's need

The assessment framework (Department of Health 2000) is a guiding map of the levels of influence impacting on a child's life. The child is located in the centre of the framework, emphasising the child-centred approach to the assessment process (see Figure 8.1).

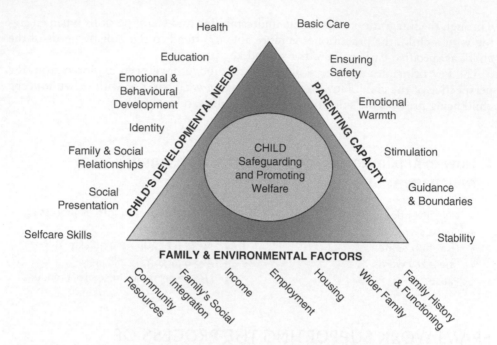

Figure 8.1   The assessment framework (Department of Health 2000)

The application of the assessment framework has been discussed in greater detail in Chapters 4 and 6. While for many the assessment may not be perceived as a framework of communication, there is an argument for considering otherwise. Each part of the assessment recognises and measures an aspect of a child's life, therefore communicating levels of risk from harm. By using the framework to guide the assessment process, the likelihood of omitting important information, for example any parental problems that may be impacting on children, can be reduced.

While many children will enter the healthcare system at different stages in their development, because of developmental health assessments and interventions or due to sustaining injury or developing illness, it is unlikely that the assessment framework will be used unless there are significant concerns of exposure to harm. Other means of recording a child's situation are therefore required in practice. Such a system would contribute to safeguarding children by ensuring appropriate, clear and accurate communication with other professionals who need to be aware of conditions underpinning an event or accident involving a child.

One framework which has received much attention in healthcare is the Situation-Background-Assessment-Recommendation tool, most often abbreviated to SBAR. The SBAR tool was developed by an American submarine officer to brief senior officers about dangerous and potentially dangerous situations. The same tool was later adapted for use within hospital settings, before evolving into the wider healthcare environment (Heinrichs et al. 2012). The SBAR has received international recognition and has been adapted for use in many different countries, including the United Kingdom. The NHS quality improvement systems recognises the SBAR as a communication tool that

Table 8.1 Description of the I-SBAR components

Structure	Description
Identify	Identify self by name, position, location.
Situation	Briefly state the problem, concern or issue. Identify the timing of events and severity.
Background	Essential background information relevant to the situation, including clinical condition and or contextual information.
Assessment	Opinion of clinical and or contextual facts.
Recommendations	What is your recommended action?

Source: Adapted from NHS Institute for Innovation and Improvement 2008

reduces communication errors, thereby contributing to quality improvement in patient care (NHS Institute for Innovation and Improvement 2008).

A major strength of this framework is its application in a multi-disciplinary context, supporting structured communication with clarity (Dayton and Henriksen 2007; European Centre of Disease Prevention and Control 2011). The framework is structured in such a manner as to provide a focus on the important aspects to be communicated or recorded. The structure standardises and prioritises information, therefore decreasing the likelihood of leaving out relevant information.

The NHS Institute for Innovation and Improvement identifies the appropriate conditions in which to use the SBAR, citing urgent and non-urgent situations, communication with other professionals and when situations have changed. It can be applied to children, young people and adults, with clinical or contextual issues indicating exposure to harm. Evaluations into the effectiveness of the SBAR are limited, with its popularity and use rising from anecdotal evidence from practice.

Identified earlier was the adaptation of the SBAR to meet differing national needs. For example, in Australia, the Situation-Background-Assessment-Recommendation tool was changed to Identify-Situation-Background-Assessment-Recommendation, referred to as I-SBAR. The inclusion of 'Identify' along with other components implies that the identity of the individual communicating to others is significant. Table 8.1 presents a description of the structured components of the SBAR as described by the NHS Institute for Innovation and Improvement (2008). In their presentation, the component labelled 'Identify' is recognised but included within the 'Situation' component. For the purpose of this text, the framework has been adapted to include all five components, as set out in the I-SBAR.

APPLYING THE I-SBAR IN PRACTICE

Take some time to read through the following case study describing a 3-year-old boy called Tom. After reading through and reflecting on Tom's reported experiences, prepare an I-SBAR report framed using the same components presented in Table 8.1. On completion of the I-SBAR, identify who needs to receive a copy of your completed report.

Tom is three years of age. He attends nursery every weekday afternoon. Tom lives with his parents and two older siblings in the nearby housing complex. He arrives at nursery every afternoon with his mother. They generally arrive on time and Tom is happy to be separated from his mother for the afternoon. One Monday afternoon, Tom arrived at nursery accompanied by an adult who was not known to the nursery staff. She stated that she was Tom's aunt who had been asked to drop Tom off at nursery on her way to town. Tom's aunt left Tom outside his classroom door, which was open. Tom's teacher found him at the entrance to the classroom on his own. She noted that as well as being on his own his lips were swollen and his front teeth were missing. As Tom was unable to immediately explain what had happened and there had not been any communication from his parents, the nursery teacher contacted the school nurse.

Exercise

You are the school nurse for the area and have been called by Tom's teacher who asks you to come to the school to assess Tom. On arrival you are taken to see Tom, who appears to be frightened and reluctant to engage. After spending some time with Tom, you eventually gain sufficient trust and Tom allows you to examine his mouth. Tom tells you that he bumped into his brother when playing at home but cannot tell you when or if he was taken to see a doctor or dentist. Your examination of Tom's mouth reveals that both sockets are dry with no visible bleeding. Tom informs you that his mouth is sore. He refused his playtime treat of a piece of fruit and juice.

The teacher provides you with background details of Tom and his family. You are informed that there have never been any concerns regarding Tom and his family and that his mother always accompanies Tom to and from the school. There are no other concerns noted by the nursery teacher.

An example of a what a completed I-SBAR relating to Tom's experiences might contain can be found in Table 8.2 at the end of this chapter.

CHALLENGES TO EFFECTIVE COMMUNICATION AND ENGAGEMENT

There a number of factors which have been identified as having the potential to impact negatively on the ability of practitioners to engage fully with children and their families and as a consequence of the safeguarding agenda.

Reflective activity

Reflecting on your own practice experiences in the clinical area, take time to consider what factors could limit the effectiveness of communication.

The need to interact with children of varying developmental abilities requires practitioners to have sophisticated verbal, non-verbal and observational skills. The ability to develop therapeutic relationships to enable conversations ranging from routine issues and health interventions to more private, intimate discussions regarding experiences of witnessing violence or exposure to abuse is central to the practice of effective communication. It cannot be assumed that children and young people, or their parents, trust all practitioners because of their professional role. Families may fear that discussing their problems with a healthcare practitioner may lead to intrusive involvement and actions by various organisations.

Children, like adults, are highly sensitive to both verbal and non-verbal methods of communication. Cossar et al. (2011) recognise that children can discriminate between practitioners who want to get to know them as individuals rather than simply get information from them. Some children may be reluctant to interact because they are fearful of upsetting their parents. It is also important to consider the possibility that in some situations children and young people may have been persuaded or coerced into concealing the truth about what has been happening to them (Scottish Government 2010). The task of relationship building can become complex and prolonged, and in some situations fails to establish sufficient meaning for the child.

Situational factors such as the physical and social environment may not be conducive to the sharing of personal and sensitive information. The physical environment can be inappropriate because of a lack of privacy, such as in a waiting area or where other people are present. A small room with no windows may seem stuffy and oppressive. The social environment can be influenced by the impact of having parents present, therefore preventing a child from discussing their experiences and feelings. A parent may use interruptions to avoid the topic or provide children with responses which would not have otherwise been made by them. It may then be difficult for a child to contradict or correct adults.

It may also be difficult for any adults involved to broach a particular topic or admit to any wrongdoing. Parents are more likely to claim any injury as the result of an accident (Roesler and Jenny 2009) whilst the child may feel unable to disclose the full extent of their concerns or may have exaggerated their worries due to the particular circumstances in which they find themselves. Dalzell and Chamberlain (2006) advise that consistencies and inconsistencies in what the child is saying should be considered alongside other accounts, as well as any presenting symptoms or injuries and relationships between the child and others.

Disclosure by a child or young person, or suspicions of abuse, may arise from a variety of sources including the child, parents, members or the public or the healthcare team. Events such as disclosure or suspicion can take place in a wide range of circumstances: opportunistic or planned encounters; during admission to the Accident & Emergency department; a hospital ward; or a routine primary care appointment with a school nurse or other healthcare professional. It is possible for such events to be viewed as a time to disclose or indeed highlight concerns about suspected abuse. For the practitioner such events can prove out of context and unexpected; however, should such events arise, they require further investigation. Children and young people's worries need to be heard and addressed.

A further limitation impacting on the effectiveness of communication are the levels of practitioner knowledge and skills. Any situation where a child selects to disclose information regarding experiences they have encountered requires sensitivity and an immediate response. Failure to respond in this manner could have a negative impact. If they are interrupted by assumptions being made which do not reflect their situation or feelings, or feel that they are being dismissed, then the likelihood of further interaction will be compromised.

For some practitioners managing situations where a child discloses information regarding an abusive experience can be difficult to handle. The use of strategies such as blocking mechanisms, for example changing the subject or ignoring what was said, although very easy to employ, can be detrimental to the child's well-being. The child or young person can feel ignored and be left feeling vulnerable (Dalzell and Chamberlain 2006).

Given some of the challenges identified when engaging children and young people and the potential for unplanned disclosure, the preparation of practitioners in engaging with children is a significant consideration.

Reflective activity

Reflecting on your experience of communicating with people in your care, can you identify the qualities of an environment that would support communication in a positive way between a child or young person and you, the practitioner?

EMERGING THEMES

Communication is the cornerstone of engaging with children and their families, and is the most common activity in healthcare settings.

The focus of communication must be child-centred and appropriate to the communication needs of every child and adult. It involves practitioners making reasonable adjustments to their practice regarding verbal, non-verbal and written communication.

An understanding of the key principles and the application of the basic skills underpinning effective communication are essential aspects of practice relating to the safeguarding agenda.

CONCLUSION

Children and young people have a right to be heard, to express themselves and to have their views taken into account. At the same time, they have the right to receive information relating to themselves in a way they understand.

In this chapter engaging with children and their parents has been examined. Key aspects of communication in the engaging process have been described. Attention has been drawn to the responsibilities of individual practitioners to be aware of the communication needs of children and their parents and to make reasonable adjustments to their practice. Finally, the assessment framework has been identified as a crucial tool in guiding the communication of every child's identified needs.

Table 8.2 I-SBAR relating to Tom's case history

Structured components	Description
Identify	Jane Brown RN, School Staff Nurse for Ashgrove Nursery
Situation	Asked to assess Tom Black, 3 years old, who attends Ashgrove Nursery. Tom was found to be missing two front teeth and has swollen lips by nursery teacher. No explanation from parents, mother not in attendance. Unsure when injury occurred. Tom unable to provide a full and accurate history of events.
Background	Tom attended nursery today 3/09/2013. His aunt left before Tom reached his classroom. His teacher noted that Tom's mouth was swollen and that his front (baby) teeth were missing. There was no bleeding. Tom said that he bumped into his brother when playing at the weekend which made his mouth sore. Parents not in attendance therefore unable to confirm events.
Assessment	*Context*: Tom lives with his parents and two siblings. Attends nursery on time every weekday afternoon, always accompanied by his mother. Never any concerns regarding Tom's development or welfare. Separation from his mother at this time does not appear to be causing him distress. *Clinical assessment*: Unsure when injury took place. On examination, front (baby) teeth missing. Sockets dry, no signs of recent bleeding. His gums are red; appear bruised and swollen, as are Tom's lips. Tom has refused refreshments which is unusual; however, he appears to have some level of pain which may explain his reluctance to eat and drink. Tom appears anxious but engages in chat.
Recommendations	Speak with Tom's mother when she calls to collect him from nursery. Establish further information regarding Tom's injury: when it happened; what happened; has Tom attended his doctor or dentist. Assess family relationships and support. Encourage Tom's mum to communicate any concerns, issues or experiences which may impact on Tom. If Tom has not yet been seen by dentists then advise that he is examined by his dentist as soon as is possible. Inform the family health visitor; family doctor and dentist. Record the I-SBAR in child records. Review Tom in one week with Tom's mother.

FURTHER READING

Brandon, M., Owers, M. and Black, J. (1999) *Learning How to Make Children Safer: An Analysis for the Welsh Office of Serious Child Abuse Cases in Wales*. Norwich: University of East Anglia/Welsh Office.

Marks-Maran, D. and Rose, P. (1997) Thinking and caring: New perspectives on reflection. In D. Marks-Maran and P. Rose (eds), *Reconstructing Nursing: Beyond Art and Science*. London: Bailliere Tindall.

Safer Healthcare (2013) *What is SBAR and What is SBAR Communication?* Littleton, CO: Safer Healthcare. Available at: www.saferhealthcare.com/sbar/what-is-sbar/ (accessed October 2012).

Scottish Government GIRFEC Team (2010) *Practice Briefing – Identifying Concern: A Guide to Implementing Getting it Right for Every Child: Messages from Pathfinders and Learning Partners*. Edinburgh: Scottish Government.

World Health Organization (2007) *Communication During Patient Hand-Overs*. Geneva: WHO Patient Safety Solutions.

REFERENCES

Beauchamp, T., Childress, J. (2001) *Principles of Biomedical Ethics*, 5th edn. Oxford: Oxford University Press.

College of Registered Nurses in Nova Scotia (2012) *Standards of Practice for Registered Nurses*. Halifax, NS: CRNNS. Available at: www.crnns.ca/documents/RNStandards.pdf (accessed July 2013).

Corby, B. (2006) *Child Abuse Towards a Knowledge Base*, 3rd edn. Milton Keynes: Open University Press.

Cossar, J., Brandon, M. and Jordan, P. (2011) '*Don't Make Assumptions': Children's and Young Peoples' Views of the Child Protection System and Messages for Change*. London: Office of the Children's Commissioner.

Cuthbert, C. and Stanley, K. (2012) All babies count: A new approach to prevention and protection for vulnerable babies. *Public Policy Research* 184: 243–247.

Dalzell, R. and Chamberlain, C. (2006) *Communicating with Children: A Two-way Process Resource Pack*. London: The National Children's Bureau.

Dayton, E. and Henriksen, K. (2007) Communication failure: Basic components, contributing factors, and the call for structure. *Joint Commission Journal on Quality and Patient Safety* 33(1): 34–47.

Department of Education and Skills (2003) *Every Child Matters*. London: The Stationery Office.

Department of Health (2000) *Framework for the Assessment of Children in Need and their Families*. London: Department of Health. Available at: http://webarchive.nationalarchives.gov.uk/+/www.dh.gov.uk/en/publicationsandstatistics/publications/publicationspolicyandguidance/dh_4003256 (accessed January 2012).

European Centre for Disease Prevention and Control (2011) *Evidence-based Methodologes for Public Health. How to Assess the Best Available Evidence When Time is Limited and I Here is Lack of Sound Evidence*. Stockholm. Technical Report. Available at: www.ecdc.europa.eu/en/publications/publications/1109_ter_evidence_based_methods_for_public_health.pdf (accessed 12 December 2013).

European Convention on Human Rights (1950) *Convention for the Protection of Human Rights and Fundamental Freedoms in Rights*. Strasbourg: European Court of Human Rights.

Heinrichs, W., Bauman, M. and Dev, P. (2012) SBAR 'flattens the hierarchy' among caregivers. *Studies in Health Technology And Informatics* 173: 175–182.

Kolucki, B. and Lemish, D. (2011) *Communicating with Children: Principles and Practices to Nurture, Inspire, Excite, Educate and Heal*. New York: UNICEF. Available at: www.unicef.org/cwc/ (accessed June 2013).

Levetown, M. (2008) Communicating with children and families: From everyday interactions to skill in conveying distressing information. *Pediatrics* 130(2): e1440–e1461.

NHS Institute for Innovation and Improvement (2008) *Quality Service and Improvement Tools: SBAR – Situation-Background-Assessment-Recommendation*. Coventry: NHS Institute for Innovation and Improvement. Available at: www.institute.nhs.uk/quality_and_service_improvement_tools/quality_and_service_improvement_tools/sbar_-_situation_-_background_-_assessment_-_recommendation/ (accessed November 2012).

Northern Ireland Assembly (2006) *Our Children and Young People – Our Shared Responsibility: The Reform Implementation Process in Child Protection Services in Northern Ireland*. Belfast: Department of Health, Social Services and Public Safety.

Roesler, T. and Jenny, C. (2009) *Beyond Munchausen Syndrome by Proxy*. Elk Grove Village, IL: American Academy of Pediatrics.

Rollnick, S., Miller, W. and Butler, C. (2008) *Motivational Interviewing in Health Care Helping Patients Change Behaviour*. London: The Guilford Press.

Scottish Executive (2005) *Getting it Right for Every Child*. Edinburgh: Scottish Executive.

Scottish Government (2010) *National Guidance for Child Protection in Scotland*. Edinburgh: Scottish Government.

Stevenson, C., Grieves, M. and Stein-Parbury, J. (2004) *Patient and Person Empowering Interpersonal Relationships in Nursing*. London: Elsevier.

Stickley, T. (2011) From SOLER to SURETY for effective non-verbal communication. *Nurse Education in Practice* 11: 395–398.

United Nations (1989) *United Nations Convention on the Rights of the Child*. Geneva: United Nations.

Welsh Assembly Government (2004) *Children and Young People: Rights to Action*. Cardiff: Welsh Assembly Government.

PART 3

FACTORS IMPACTING ON PRACTICE

9

RESPONDING TO DOMESTIC ABUSE IN THE LIVES OF CHILDREN

SANDRA RODWELL

CHAPTER SUMMARY

Domestic abuse is an important gendered, public health issue, which has continued to gain prominence in the national and international policy arena. The nature and extent of violence and abuse perpetrated by men towards women, however manifest, has prompted some to make comparisons with torture (Stanko 1997; World Health Organization 1997). There is general agreement that men are most likely to perpetrate the most serious forms of domestic abuse involving extreme violence and murder. The cost to individuals, communities and society of what was previously considered to be a private affair is now publicly expressed in both economic and health terms, culminating in an infringement of the human rights of women and children.

In relation to children who live with domestic abuse, the impact on their well-being and the potential risk of direct harm means they are considered as children 'in need' and potentially at risk of significant harm. All practitioners have an increasing role to play in the area of primary, secondary and tertiary prevention with respect to safeguarding and protecting the child (Royal College of Nursing 2007).

The response of practitioners to domestic abuse in the lives of their clients will in part be influenced by the individual practitioners' understanding of a particular situation. This understanding will not only be shaped by personal beliefs, values and experiences, but also by professional codes of conduct and the managerial and organisational environment in which they practice. The approach specified as appropriate through the dominant discourse within which domestic abuse is situated will also have some influence (Woodtli 2000; Tarlier 2004).

This chapter begins by considering domestic abuse in the lives of children. A discussion of the potential impact on practice of how this social phenomenon is named and understood is also presented. The impact of the healthcare environment, for example national and local policies, and how this shapes the focus of care is then discussed. This chapter concludes by drawing on the findings of the author's doctoral study (Rodwell 2008), providing an illustrative account of four key aspects of practice identified by study participants as either facilitating or constraining the response of practitioners working in a community setting to children living with domestic abuse. The client relationship and the redistribution of power, the moral and ethical dilemmas facing practitioners, the emotional aspects of practice and the role of support and supervision are discussed.

AIMS OF THIS CHAPTER

The overall aim of this chapter is to provide the reader with an opportunity to consider critically the factors which may impact on their response as a practitioner to children living with domestic abuse.

Learning outcomes

After reading this chapter and following a period of reflection the reader will be able to:

- Develop a better understanding of the way children and young people experience domestic abuse.
- Critically reflect on the potential impact on children and young people of living with domestic abuse.
- Analyse critically the link between domestic abuse and child abuse.
- Consider critically the different factors that could influence their practice in response to domestic abuse in the lives of children.
- Develop a better understanding of the role of support and supervision.

Key words

child; children in need of protection; community setting; domestic abuse; feminism; practice; support and supervision

DOMESTIC ABUSE IN THE LIVES OF CHILDREN

The prevalence of domestic abuse in the lives of children

It is not possible to accurately identify the number of children living with domestic abuse. It has been estimated that in England and Wales at least 750,000 children witness domestic abuse and that three-quarters of the children on the Child Protection Register live in households where domestic abuse occurs (Department of Health 2003). In Scotland it has been estimated that 100,000 children (one in ten) live in families where domestic abuse is a feature (Blamey et al. 2002). More recent statistics suggest that on average across the United Kingdom one in seven (14.2 per cent) children and young people under the age of 18 will have lived with domestic abuse at some point in their childhood (Radford et al. 2011).

Although limited, the available estimates have prompted some to describe the situation of children and young people as a 'chronic social problem' (Humphreys 2006: 20). Recognising domestic abuse as a situation which poses a risk to children reinforces the need for practitioners to understand the dynamics of this social phenomenon.

Children's experiences of living with domestic abuse

Children experience domestic abuse in various ways. It has been recognised for some time that domestic abuse may start or escalate during pregnancy (Mezey and Bewley 1997; Stanley 2011). Being subjected to domestic abuse at this time puts both the physical and mental well-being of the mother and fetus at risk.

Children may be in the same room when an incident is taking place, hear events as they unfold in another room, be aware of physical signs of injury to an adult or damage to property. Situations where children have witnessed their mother being sexually assaulted have also been reported (McGee 2000). Children may become involved in the abuse accidentally while trying to intervene, be used as a pawn to bargain or threaten, or become the direct subject of abuse, which may be physical, sexual, emotional or a combination of these (Mullender et al. 2002; Holt et al. 2008). Children may continue to experience the impact of domestic abuse during contact visits even though they no longer live with the abusive adult (Stanley 2011).

Children from poorer socioeconomic areas may be exposed to community violence as part of everyday life (Osofsky 1999; Herrenkohl et al. 2008). Violent images are also readily accessible through television, videos, DVDs and music. Osofsky (1999) carried out a systematic review of studies reporting on the effects on children of three types of violence: domestic abuse, community violence and media violence. In his final analysis Osofsky concluded that in order to appreciate the impact on children of exposure to violence, in whichever form it took, it was important to take account of the child's wider environment.

The potential impact on children of living with domestic abuse

The behavioural and emotional impact on children of living with domestic abuse is identified throughout the literature (Edleson 1999; Hester et al. 2000; McGee 2000; Mullender et al. 2002; Holt et al. 2008; Herrenkohl et al. 2008; Stanely 2011). Comparisons with the experiences of individuals suffering from post traumatic stress disorder have been made (Wolak and Finkelhor 1998; Osofsky 1999; Hester et al. 2000).

Children and young people themselves have reported experiencing feelings of guilt, confusion, sadness, self-blame, depression, anxiety and loss (Wolak and Finkelhor 1998; Edleson 1999; McGee 2000; Hester at al. 2000; Mullender et al. 2002). A link between the recent witnessing of domestic abuse and subsequent violent behaviour is also reported, alongside poor verbal, motor and cognitive skills (Edleson 1999). Higher levels of internalised responses have also been reported, which can manifest themselves in the form of sleep disturbance, bed-wetting and nightmares (Wolak and Finkelhor 1998; Edleson 1999).

However, there is some research which suggests that there are a number of factors which impact on the response of a child. The age of the child, their relationship with the abuser and abused, the forms of violence witnessed, the extent of their involvement and the availability of support, both within the family and from others, are identified as possible dimensions that can influence the outcomes for a child. Individual characteristics pertaining to the child itself may also impact on their response to the situation (Cleaver et al. 1999; Holt et al. 2008; Stanley 2011). How gender impacts on the responses of children remains poorly researched (Humphreys 2006).

One study which consulted children from a range of backgrounds and experiences across England and Wales found that children considered psychological and emotional abuse to be worse than physical violence. Living in fear of further violence was also considered to be very stressful, as was the inability to control what was happening (McGee 2000).

Domestic abuse, child abuse and neglect

The psychological and or physical effects of domestic abuse impact on a parent's ability to parent effectively (Hester et al. 2000; McGee 2000; Stanley 2011). However, studies which have explored the impact on parenting have mainly focused on the negative effects on the mother's parenting capacity, without giving full consideration to the circumstances in which parenting is taking place (Hartley 2004). The parenting skills of the father as the most likely perpetrator of domestic abuse are left unchallenged.

Increased levels of child abuse have been shown to occur in families where domestic abuse was an issue, as opposed to families where it was not. However, the rates of child abuse carried out by either fathers (as perpetrators of domestic abuse) or mothers (as victims of domestic abuse) appears to vary depending on the forms of behaviour that are considered as child abuse. Studies that focus on severe physical abuse towards children report higher rates of fathers being responsible for the abuse. However, if child abuse encompasses a wider number of apparently less severe forms of abuse such as pushing or slapping, then mothers are more likely to be the ones to abuse their children (Hartley 2004).

Children living with domestic abuse have given different accounts of their relationship with their mother. Some children have talked about feeling closer as a consequence of the violence and abuse. For others their relationship is said to be poor, with children holding their mothers responsible for the violence and abuse they (the mother and the child) are living with (McGee 2000).

The co-occurrence of domestic abuse and physical and sexual abuse of children was first established in the United States as early as the 1960s (Hester et al. 2000). Within the United Kingdom studies focused on child protection have highlighted the link between child abuse and neglect and domestic abuse (Hester et al. 2000). In the most extreme cases children are killed in families where there is domestic abuse (Hester et al. 2000).

An association between the extent of physical violence towards a female partner and the physical abuse of children within that relationship has been established, initially through studies carried out in America (Edleson 1999). Having reviewed a number of studies, Edleson (2002) noted that while the setting and the samples involved in the studies were different, the overlap between domestic abuse and child abuse was apparent. However, despite the greater risk to this particular group, children living with domestic abuse are not routinely assessed for child abuse and neglect (Wolak and Finkelhor 1998). While not all children living with domestic abuse are adversely affected by their experiences, domestic abuse has been recognised as an indicator of child abuse and neglect (Powell 2003; Holt et al. 2008).

Further and more detailed analysis of the findings from the first ever prevalence study of the experiences of children and young people in relation to abuse and neglect carried out in the United Kingdom has been reported on by Cawson (2002). In this second report, the author gives an account of the reported co-occurrence of physical and sexual child abuse and domestic abuse. Eight out of ten participants who said they had suffered from serious physical abuse also reported having experienced domestic abuse. Of the 27 who reported having been subjected to sexual abuse, 21 also reported domestic abuse. Findings such as these demonstrate that domestic abuse and child abuse are not mutually exclusive.

The long-term impact of living with domestic abuse

Studies looking at the long-term impact on children and young people witnessing domestic abuse and being subject to personal violence have suggested a possible association with depression, violent and criminal behaviour and the occurrence of domestic abuse in adulthood (Wolak and Finkehor 1998; Edelson 1999; Russell et al. 2010). However, the sampling strategy adopted in retrospective studies may introduce an element of bias as only adults with particular difficulties may be consulted about their childhood experiences. For example, an association between adult depression and childhood exposure to domestic abuse may appear more significant than it actually is due to the bias introduced in the sampling process where only adults with depression are asked about their childhood experiences. The retrospective nature of the data may also introduce an element of bias.

The findings from research suggest the need for caution against the assumption that all children will be adversely affected in the long-term by their childhood experiences. The observation that different children respond in different ways emphasises the interconnected nature of the factors that can have a protective effect in some instances or intensify the experience in others (Holt et al. 2008; Russell et al. 2010). One of the key messages to emerge is the need to talk about associations rather than assume a cause-and-effect outcome. The knowledge that the potential impact on children of living with domestic abuse is not linear highlights the importance of practitioners adopting assessment processes that take account of the interaction of multiple factors at a number of levels. It also underlines the importance of being aware of the wider evidence base while considering each case on its own merits and not just following a set path.

Key points

- Children experience domestic abuse both directly and indirectly.
- The emotional and physical needs of children living with domestic abuse may not be fully met.
- Focusing on the mother as the main source of support may not benefit the child or the mother.
- Living with domestic abuse is an important indicator that children are at risk of harm.
- Practitioners need to be aware of the co-occurrence of child abuse, neglect and domestic abuse.
- Practitioners need to be alert to the possibility that a child may be subjected to more than one form of abuse, for example the wider environment they live in.
- Children may continue to experience the impact of domestic abuse although they no longer live with the abusive adult.
- There are a number of mediating factors in the lives of individual children which influence the long-term impact of living with domestic abuse.

Reflective activity

After reading the information in the above section, identify and read a selection of professional guidelines as well as national and local policies and procedures relating to domestic abuse in the lives of children.

Reflecting on their content, do you feel your selected documents provide enough guidance and support for practitioners?

NAMING THE EXPERIENCE

In the past there has been a debate in the literature around the adequacy of the terminology used to describe domestic abuse. Different labels may impact differently on the perceptions held by the public, professionals and politicians as to the nature of violence and abuse against women and whether it should be considered a private or a public affair (Featherstone and Trinder 1997; Stanley 1997; Dobash and Dobash 1998; Jouriles et al. 2000).

Labels such as 'domestic abuse', 'domestic violence', 'battered women', 'intimate partner violence', 'violence towards women by known men', 'partner violence' and 'family violence' are all used throughout the literature. However, these labels are misleading in describing not only the relationship between partners and ex-partners but also the severity, nature, extent and intent of the violence and abuse. Labels such as 'partner violence' may suggest behaviour which is reciprocal, while the use of the term 'domestic' suggests that this phenomenon occurs only within the home environment, reinforcing the belief that it is a private affair.

The use of terms such as 'victim' and 'survivor' are also questioned in the literature. Classifying women in relation to their experience of domestic abuse and by association with abusive men is considered to perpetuate the societal view of men holding power over women. Women are then portrayed as passive recipients of abusive and violent behaviour. This portrayal belies the varied experiences of women in relation to violence and abuse and the diversity of women themselves (Chung 2001–2002). The focus on women as victims of domestic abuse is also seen as a barrier to women voicing concern over their own behaviour, their experiences of abuse by other women and the potential for abusive behaviour towards their children (Featherstone and Trinder 1997; Fitzroy 2001).

Key point

- The terminology we use to describe a phenomenon can influence the way practitioners respond in practice to women, children and men.

Reflective activity

Take some time to reflect on the language you use when referring to perpetrators and those living with violence and abuse, then consider the following questions:

- What factors influence your choice of terminology?
- Does the language you use reflect your understanding of the phenomenon?
- Does the language you use impact on your practice?
- Are there changes you now feel you could make to the language you use?

FEMINIST THEORY AND THE POLITICAL AGENDA

Over time the experiences of women as told by women themselves, or advocates on their behalf (e.g. organisations such as Women's Aid), have emerged as the dominant voice in relation to domestic abuse. Women's experiences have informed public, political and legal arenas nationally and internationally as to the nature, extent and cause of domestic abuse (Featherstone and Trinder 1997; Hawkins and Humes 2002).

It is likely that the approach adopted by grassroots women's groups, set up for women by women, has been underpinned by the developing feminist theories of the early 1970s. These groups defined domestic abuse as a manifestation of a patriarchal society where men exercise their power over women and children whilst maintaining their economic, social and cultural dominance (Tong 1989; Featherstone and Trinder 1997). However, not strands of feminist theories have something to say about men's violence towards women (Tong 1989). The meaning and experiences of domestic abuse for women from different cultures, social groups and of different colour is relatively unexplored (Greenan 2004). Feminist theories are also limited in their ability to account for female violence in same-sex relationships (Fitzroy 2001; Perilla et al. 2003).

As domestic abuse has gained prominence within the political arena both nationally and internationally, the situation of women and children as those most likely to be subjected to domestic abuse has dominated the agenda. The estimated cost of domestic abuse, both financially and in health terms, has influenced the deployment of resources. National and regional governments within the United Kingdom have focused on the development of services aimed at supporting women and children. Nonetheless, the extent to which such organisations can or should represent all women is open to question given the relatively small proportion of women living with domestic abuse who use the services provided by organisations such as Women's Aid (Radford and Hester 2001). Assuming that one particular perspective provides a privileged insight into a particular phenomenon has the potential to limit the scope for a robust analysis and appropriate action to bring about change (Atkinson 1997).

Adults and children whose experiences of domestic abuse do not conform to the dominant pattern, such as adults in same-sex relationships and men in heterosexual relationships, may find it hard to access support. The needs of children living in situations where domestic abuse is an issue may be overlooked. Conversely, practice which adopts a more inclusive approach by acknowledging women's violence, looking more critically at the violence of men or is seen to separate the needs of women and children, may serve to favour men and further penalise women.

> ## Key points
>
> - The situation of women and children as those most likely to be subjected to domestic abuse dominates the political agenda and the response of practitioners.

- An unintended consequence of the focus on gender is that adults and children whose experiences of domestic abuse do not conform to the dominant pattern may find it hard to access support.
- A more inclusive approach which acknowledges women's violence and looks more critically at the violence of men, or is seen to separate the needs of women and children, may serve to favour men and further penalise women.

Reflective activity

Reflecting on the section above, consider how the focus on the gendered nature of domestic abuse impacts on the response of practitioners to domestic abuse in the lives of children.

Did you consider children living in families who experience domestic abuse and who do not conform to the dominant pattern?

THE HEALTHCARE CONTEXT

Providing care closer to home

Aimed at governments, health and development workers and the world community, the World Health Organization (1978) stressed the importance of a co-ordinated approach to health by all relevant sectors, inclusive of health and social care. Central to the approach set out in the Alma Alta declaration is the involvement of individuals and communities in identifying their health needs and the development and delivery of appropriate services within the communities where people live (WHO 1978). Within the United Kingdom the principle of providing healthcare in or close to clients' homes has gathered momentum since the NHS and Community Care Act in 1990.

Working within a community setting gives practitioners the opportunity to work with vulnerable groups such as children, babies, women during pregnancy and the postnatal period, and the elderly. Potential access to diverse groups and the apparent acceptability of their involvement underlines the key role practitioners have in addressing a number of important public health priorities in line with legislative and policy initiatives (Sines 2001; Kelly and Symonds 2003). Based on the premise that early support for children and families may prevent the risk of significant harm to children, all nurses, midwives and other health professionals are encouraged to be alert to potential stressors which impact on the health and welfare of clients and their families. Domestic abuse is one such stressor.

A public health approach

Public health initiatives aimed at preventing ill-health take place at a primary, secondary and tertiary level. However, the distinction between each level may be blurred

(Elliot et al. 2001). Primary prevention initiatives focus on raising awareness amongst the general population about a particular area of concern. The aim of this approach also highlights the steps that individuals, professionals and organisations can take to keep the general population well. Within the context of domestic abuse, the universal service provided by health visitors to all families with children under school age provides an opportunity for primary prevention through support and education for all parents.

Secondary prevention is focused on early prevention within the context of populations known to be vulnerable to a particular condition, event or circumstance. This approach increases the opportunity to develop early interventions. Initiatives aimed at developing a proactive approach by all practitioners to identifying domestic abuse in the lives of their clients increase the opportunity to identify and respond to the needs of children, including the need for protection (Royal College of Nursing 2007).

Initiatives developed within the context of tertiary prevention are aimed at managing the impact of a particular condition, event or set of circumstances in already known cases. Once domestic abuse is known to be a concern within the lives of clients, be they adults or children, practitioners need to take appropriate action. An appropriate response may include giving information, education and referral to an agency providing support for women (as the most likely parent to be abused) and children.

Advocating for better services for vulnerable groups, inclusive of issues about access, also forms part of an appropriate action. As well as working with individuals and their families, practitioners working in a community setting can contribute to community based initiatives.

Health visitors, through the provision of a universal home visiting service, have historically adopted a public health focused approach to families with young children (Sines 2001). However, the present emphasis on care within a community setting and public health may present new ways of working for practitioners from other branches of nursing.

The changing context of care presents practitioners with the need to manage the potentially competing agendas of organisational and professional priorities and those of clients themselves. Having reviewed the changing context of care, Sines states that these changes challenge 'traditional boundaries and working practices for all staff and demand a deconstruction of previously defended allegiances to unidisciplinary patterns of working' (2001: 10).

Key points

- Working within a community setting gives practitioners the opportunity to work with vulnerable and diverse groups, inclusive of those who may have little contact with other services.
- The apparent acceptability of the involvement of practitioners underlines the key role they have in addressing a number of important public health priorities.

- The changing context of care presents practitioners with the need to manage the potentially competing agendas of organisational and professional priorities and those of their clients.

Reflective activity

List all of the ethical challenges you can think of that practitioners face when working in a community setting in their response to domestic abuse in the lives of children.

What role do you envisage for practitioners working in a community setting in response to domestic abuse in the lives of children?

RESPONDING TO DOMESTIC ABUSE IN PRACTICE

With reference to the author's doctoral study (Rodwell 2008), this section explores key aspects of practice identified as having the potential to either facilitate or constrain the response of practitioners working in a community setting to children living with domestic abuse. Practitioners working in a community setting were the key informants. A sequential mixed-method design influenced by the Delphi technique was applied to the study and comprised individual face-to-face interviews and two self-completion questionnaires. Through their collective responses, participants outlined an important role for practitioners in response to children living with domestic abuse.

The role of practitioners

Participants in Rodwell's (2008) doctoral study identified four key elements for practitioners working with children living with domestic violence: advocacy; identification; assessment of need; and referral to other sources of support or child protection as appropriate. At the same time, however, participants raised questions as to the feasibility of all practitioners working in a community setting fulfilling such a role. While practitioners may have concerns for the well-being and safety of children living with domestic abuse, the findings from this doctoral study suggest that the needs of children living with domestic abuse continue to be marginalised. This doctoral study identified a gap between the intentions set out in policy and the reality of practice. As practitioners engage with the wider health and social issues their actions are both enhanced and constrained by a number of factors.

For practitioners working in a community setting the context is far more than the geographical location of care and domestic abuse as a specific and discrete event. The wider health and social circumstances of the client and the nurse–client relationship forms part of the context. The moral-ethical dilemmas and the emotional aspects of practice may also shape their actions. Adopting a child-centred response to an adult-focused problem is challenged by the context in which care is delivered.

The nurse–client relationship and the redistribution of power

The ideology of partnership working and the nurse–client relationship are central tenets of a nursing process which is focused on the delivery of person-centred holistic care (Carr et al. 2001: Tschudin 2003). Working in partnership with clients necessarily involves consideration being given to the re-distribution of power as practitioners move from 'doing to' and 'for' to 'doing with' (Carr et al. 2001; Gallant et al. 2002). The overall aim of this approach is to support the client to find ways of managing their situation (Gallant et al. 2002; Hyland 2002; Brown et al. 2006). The practice of practitioners has to take account of the redistribution of power and the dilemmas this may create.

During the doctoral study (Rodwell 2008) some participants described the process of developing a relationship with their clients as one that took time and was based on trust. Participants talked about 'being there for the family' and 'allowing families time'. The nurse–client relationship described by most participants concurred with the process of partnership outlined by Gallant et al. (2002) where clients are viewed as active participants and equal partners. This philosophy is implicit in government policies specific to domestic abuse. However, as was evidenced through the response of participants in the doctoral study, aspects of partnership working and the nurse–client relationship could both enhance and constrain the practice of practitioners in response to adults and children living with domestic abuse.

As a consequence of the nurse–client relationship clients may reveal different aspects of their lives, including issues around domestic abuse. However, within the complexity of the everyday lives of clients, as described by some participants in the doctoral study, domestic abuse was not necessarily high on the list of concerns for either the practitioner or the client. The focus of nursing care, for example substance misuse, mental health or the physical care of children with life-limiting conditions, was presented by some as drawing boundaries around the extent to which practitioners could proactively engage in the domestic abuse agenda. Some participants also spoke about becoming almost immune to some of the circumstances people lived with, particularly when other serious issues were impacting on an individual person or family (Rodwell 2008).

Participants in the doctoral study talked about 'a fine line'. This 'fine line' threaded its way through the collective responses and appeared to represent the tension and dilemmas nurses face as they balance a number of competing and contradictory priorities. One such contributory factor was the issue of agenda setting. Situations where clients had chosen not to engage with the nurse in relation to the violence and abuse within their lives were recounted. The situation for practitioners could be further complicated by the difficulties experienced by individual practitioners in raising and addressing the issue of domestic abuse with parents and the potential impact on children living with domestic abuse. While working in partnership with adult clients – or families with children who require nursing care – facilitates shared decision making, it does not exempt practitioners from their professional responsibility towards children.

Also woven through the accounts of participants was a narrative encapsulated in the phrase 'it all depends'. 'It all depends' reflected the sense of helplessness some participants felt as they considered the role of practitioners and the limited impact practitioners could realistically have on the situation for children. This stemmed from the assessment that practitioners were ultimately unable to control the environment in which children live. The interaction between these two narratives captured the tension between the rhetoric of policy and the day-to-day experience of practitioners.

A discussion paper presented by Hanafin (1998) cautions against unrealistic expectation when it comes to the role of nurses working in a community setting and the protection of children, specifically in situations where child neglect and abuse have been identified. The key concern raised by Hanafin was the mismatch between the actual role nurses can undertake and the expectations of others, particularly those charged with providing child protection services.

The accounts of some participants in the doctoral study described situations which presented a number of moral-ethical dilemmas.

Moral-ethical dilemmas

Moral-ethical dilemmas are defined as situations where a nurse may be presented with conflicting moral claims or loyalties. Within the context of partnership working and the nurse–client relationship, another source of uncertainty was the apparent tension between the ethical principles of beneficence (to do good), non-maleficence (to do no harm) and the duty of care towards children (Rodwell 2008). These dilemmas raise questions as to how concepts such as individual choice, equity, respect and confidentiality translate in practice when working with a family where a mother is subject to violent and abusive behaviour and the client may be either the perpetrator, the victim or a child.

An example of the dilemmas evident in the response of some participants in the doctoral study was a situation where empathy with the client and concern over the unintended consequences of involving others could lead to a cautious response to children (Rodwell 2008). One participant spoke about 'giving the mother another chance' in situations where there were no obvious child protection issues. However, this participant was also aware that this was not necessarily the right response for the child. While practitioners may be aware that supporting the mother does not necessarily mean that the situation for the child will improve, their relationships with the non-abusing parent may interfere with their role as an advocate for the child.

Through her theoretical exploration of the relationships between patient autonomy and patient advocacy, Hyland (2002) warns against an over-emphasis on autonomy, particularly in situations where the client themselves or another is then harmed. Hyland states that 'nurses may stand accused of negligence, by act or omission' (2002: 481). This is particularly pertinent to the subject of this chapter as partnership working, the nurse–client relationship and autonomy for the client appear to challenge the development of an appropriate response to children living with domestic abuse. In some circumstances, the role practitioners could adopt in response to children becomes lost among their concerns about acting inappropriately given the difficult circumstances already impacting on individual clients and families.

Drawing on a case study based on her earlier experiences as a student nurse, Pask (2001) explored the concept of moral agency in nursing. The question driving her discussion was 'are we justified in holding nurses responsible for their behaviour in situations of patient care'? Pask concludes that 'what is needed is a moral climate that sustains nurses as they attempt to shape their behaviour and to develop their emotions as they respond to the demands that are put upon them in today's world of healthcare' (2001: 51). The emotional aspect of working with families where domestic abuse is an issue and the moral-ethical dilemmas nurses face can lead to incorrect decisions about how to respond, which, while not deliberately neglectful of children, may prove to be just that. The 'fear' of getting it wrong or making things worse may lead to inaction. Some of the responses of participants in the doctoral study constructed a picture of practitioners watching and waiting for something to happen before they could act (Rodwell 2008).

Some participants expressed feelings of anger, frustration, sadness and helplessness as they discussed their involvement with families where domestic abuse had been an issue. These feelings were in response to the choices clients made and the extent to which nurses could influence the outcomes and the situations that some clients lived with.

The emotional aspects of practice

The emotional aspects of caring work can be undervalued or ignored by practitioners themselves, organisations and society as a whole due to the association this form of labour has with the work of women and the private rather than the public sphere of life (Hochschild 1983; Phillips 1996; Staden 1998; Gray 2002; Mazhindu 2003).

The experiences recounted by participants in the doctoral study (Rodwell 2008) reflected the concept of 'emotional labour' identified by Hochschild (1983). Hochschild defined 'emotional labour' as a form of labour which required the labourer to manage or suppress their own emotions in order to enhance the well-being of another. Three criteria were identified as defining the situation in which emotional labour is performed. The experiences of practitioners working in a community setting meet these three criteria.

The first criterion is that the work or labour involves direct contact with people (Hochschild 1983). Practitioners working in a community setting not only have direct contact with clients, they are also made aware of the different circumstances which may impact on a client's life. There is then the potential to become involved with different aspects of the client's life. The second criterion refers to the situation where working directly with people requires the labourer or worker to respond in such a way that enhances the well-being of another (Hochschild 1983). This particular criterion is at the heart of nursing practice and the holistic philosophy of care. The third criterion is that the employer can direct the focus of the emotional work (Hochschild 1983). Professional standards and national and local policies and guidelines direct the work of practitioners. To summarise, performing emotional labour involves the worker in giving something personal of themselves.

In the doctoral study the perception was that some nurses chose to ignore domestic abuse in the lives of women and children. 'Putting up the shutters' and ignoring the impact of domestic abuse in the lives of children maybe a protective mechanism (Rodwell 2008). The apparent disinterest of some practitioners may be a consequence of doubt, anxiety and the emotional and moral-ethical dilemmas they face. The experience of uncertainty appeared to result in a reactive rather than a proactive approach to the needs of children and an emphasis on physical signs of harm (Rodwell 2008).

Within the context of the doctoral study some participants talked about the skill and sensitivity required in addressing domestic abuse and in particular domestic abuse in the lives of children. The cost to the nurse of performing emotional labour was acknowledged by some participants, and evidenced by the call for support and supervision (Rodwell 2008). At the same time some participants also talked about controlling their emotions, which were seen to get in the way of being professional. Such an approach involved standing back and making an objective assessment of the circumstances in which children were living (Rodwell 2008). However, Benner (1984) notes that a distant observer may miss subtle nuances.

Support and supervision

Participants in the doctoral study saw formal and informal support and supervision as a mechanism for encouraging reflective practice. It was stated that through this process nurses could access peer review, advice, guidance and support. However, an apparent lack of support and supervision structures was also reported by participants (Rodwell 2008). At the same time it was recognised that not all practitioners actively engaged in formal or informal support mechanisms. The potential for community practitioners to practice without direct access to both formal and informal support and supervision (either through choice or limited availability), raises questions at both an individual practitioner level and at an organisational level if nurses' practice, which involves emotional labour, is neither supported nor challenged in a robust, systematic and positive way.

The need for support and supervision which ran through this doctoral study mirrored those reported on by Lister and Crisp (2005). They carried out a study aimed at exploring the views and experiences of community nurses and nurse managers in relation to clinical supervision and child protection. The authors found that some viewed clinical supervision in a negative light. The nursing culture in the area of child protection appeared to equate supervision with not coping. Formal structures of supervision were also considered by some as a managerial tool for 'monitoring bad practice' (2005: 65). The authors state that for supervision to be effective, it needs to take place within a trusting relationship. Overall, however, participants' responses also suggested that previous cautionary views about supervision were changing (Lister and Crisp 2005). That said, they conclude that both the nurses and nurse managers emphasised the need for formal supervisory and supportive structures in relation to community nurses' responsibility for protecting children.

EMERGING THEMES

Practitioners need to be supported to explore their own views and beliefs in relation to domestic abuse, and specifically domestic abuse in the lives of children.

Practitioners should feel safe enough to reflect on their actions and critically consider what they may have done differently.

CASE STUDY

James is a Learning Disability nurse and has worked in the community as part of the Learning Disability team for the last three years. His role is to care for children and young people. One client James has regular contact with is Karen. Karen is four years of age and has Down's syndrome as well as a congenital heart defect. Karen is an affectionate and chatty child who is enthusiastic about using Makaton in order to make herself understood. Karen has regular sessions with the speech and language therapist. It is normal for Karen's father David to accompany her when she visits the clinic. Karen has missed the last two appointments and the therapist has contacted James.

James has developed a good rapport with Karen's dad. Karen's mother Tracy is rarely present when he makes a home visit. Over the past few visits, James has noted a change in Karen's behaviour and appearance. She appears withdrawn and no longer approaches him on arrival. Less care had been taken over Karen's appearance. He also noted that Karen's father was less interactive with James.

Having spoken with the speech and language therapist, James decides to visit the family. James notes that Tracy is present but appears to remain in the background, though watchful. The home atmosphere appeared tense and James had a sense that all was not well but could not identify the problem. He asked Karen's dad how things were going and was repeatedly informed that everything was 'OK'. James asked about the missed appointments and was told that they had family staying with them and that they would be along to the next scheduled appointment with the speech and language therapist. James knew that David understood the implications of Karen's condition. Reflecting on his findings and uncertainties, James decided to discuss Karen's situation with his supervisor.

Reflective activity

Reflecting on the identified changes to Karen, can you identify the possible causes?

During his meeting with his supervisor, James raises his concerns regarding his findings about Karen. James explained that although her clinical condition appeared unchanged, he was concerned about the changes in her behaviour and appearance. James also raised the issue of his perceptions regarding a feeling of tension within the home on his last few visits and the missed appointments with the speech and language therapist.

The supervisor asked James what he thought were the reasons for such changes. After some consideration, James suggested that perhaps there was something like abuse going on:

Supervisor: What made you think of that?

James: Well, I don't know, just a feeling. On the surface David was his usual self but he seemed a bit edgy and not as chatty as usual.

Supervisor: OK, but what about the mum?

James: Karen's mum is never really around. However, she has been at home more recently but she never really gets involved.

Supervisor: OK, what are you considering now?

James: Well, I don't know. Could Karen's dad be abusing her mum?

Supervisor: What makes you think of that? Is there an alternative reason then?

James: Well, from what I have seen of her, I could not see any obvious bruising or other injuries. But you know, now that I come to think about it, I did see sort of small, what looked like burns on the dad's arms. Do you really think that she is abusing Karen's dad?

Supervisor: What evidence makes you think of that?

Reflective activity

Reflecting on Karen's home environment, what signs suggest that abuse is taking place?

James sat for a minute reflecting on all the points he had noted regarding the changes with Karen and her family. James thought that Karen's change in behaviour could very possibly result from witnessing abuse or violence between her parents. But how could Karen's mother be abusing her dad? Isn't it more likely to be the other way round? James stated this to his supervisor, who agreed, but added that in a small number of cases it is the man who is being abused. Further discussion followed:

James: What happens now?
Supervisor: Well, what do you think needs to happen?
James: It is important that Karen remains at home with her family.
Supervisor: But is she safe with James in her present environment?
James: Well, yes, I think her mother would not harm Karen!
Supervisor: What do you think has changed Karen's behaviour? Why is she so with-
             drawn? And is it right that she remains in that environment when she
             could be at risk of harm?
James: I suppose you are right!
Supervisor: Doing nothing is an action in itself, and may add to the risks to Karen.
James: Oh yes! I see what you mean. OK, what happens next? What do I need
             to do now?

The supervisor directs James to make sure that all his observations of Karen and her family are recorded in detail, including the supervisory session. He then strongly advises James to familiarise himself with the child safeguarding and protection policy. At this point the supervisor reminded James that he was not the only practitioner involved with Karen and that others had possibly also noted similar changes. James was directed to contact the local child protection team to advise them of his observations and concerns.

A referral was made to the local Child Protection Service. A formal investigation was undertaken. During this period Karen's mother left the family home.

During the next few supervision sessions James expressed his concern over the possibility that he had been responsible for breaking up Karen's home as her mum had left the family. He also stated that he had considered that the abuse could have been going on for some time. The supervisor informed James that he had taken the correct action in reporting his findings.

James continued working closely with Karen and her father in order to support David in helping Karen understand what was happening. James also helped David develop strategies to respond to Karen's confusion which was expressed through her behaviour.

It is important for practitioners like James to understand the need to take action regardless of how much doubt there might be about what is going on. A small piece of the jigsaw contributes to the larger picture. Practitioners are not alone.

CONCLUSION

This chapter has highlighted the complex and sometimes contradictory context in which practitioners working in a community setting respond to domestic abuse in the lives of children. A number of factors which can either enhance or constrain practice have been explored. Attention has been drawn to the continuing possibility of an inconsistent and reactive response by practitioners to children living with domestic abuse despite an increase in the levels of professional and political concern. The importance of practitioners engaging in the support and supervision process has been highlighted. The case study also demonstrated the need for a multi-disciplinary, multi-agency approach which follows the local safeguarding policies and protocols. While not deliberately neglectful of children, the decision taken by individual practitioners may prove to be just that.

Reflective activity

Having read this chapter, take time to consider your reaction to the discussions you have been encouraged to reflect on.

- What did you find helpful?
- How do you feel?

FURTHER READING

Abrahams, H. (2007) *Supporting Women after Domestic Violence: Loss, Trauma and Recovery.* London: Jessica Kingsley.

Burkhardt, M. A. and Nathaniel, A. K. (2002) *Ethics and Issues in Contemporary Nursing*, 2nd edn. Albany, NY: Delmar.

Gorin, S. (2004) *Understanding What Children Say: Children's Experiences of Domestic Violence, Parental Substance Misuse and Parental Health Problems.* London: National Children's Bureau.

McLaughlin, J. (2003) *Feminist Social and Political Theory: Contemporary Debates and Dialogues.* New York. Palgrave Macmillan.

Walby, S. (2004) *The Cost of Domestic Violence.* London: Women and Equality Unit. Retrieved from: www.womenandequalityunit.gov.uk (accessed November 2004).

REFERENCES

Atkinson, P. (1997) Narrative turn or blind alley? *Qualitative Health Research* 7(3): 325–344.

Benner, P. (1984) *From Novice to Expert: Excellence and Power in Clinical Nursing Practice.* Menlo Park, CA: Addison-Wesley.

Blamey, A., Hanlon, P., Judge, K. and Muririe, J. (2002) *Health Inequalities in the New Scotland*. Glasgow: Public Health Institute for Scotland.

Brown, D., McWilliam, C. and Ward-Griffin, C. (2006) Client-centred empowering partnering in nursing. *Journal of Advanced Nursing* 53(2): 160–168.

Carr, S., Bell, B., Pearson, P. and Watson, D. (2001) To be sure or not to be sure: Concepts of uncertainty and risk in the construction of community nursing practice. *Primary Health Care and Development* 2: 223–233.

Cawson, P. (2002) *Child Maltreatment in the Family: The Experience of a National Sample of Young People*. London: NSPCC.

Chung, D. (2001–2002) Questioning domestic violence orthodoxies: Challenging the social construction of women as victims and as being responsible for stopping male violence. *Women Against Violence* 11: 7–15.

Cleaver, H., Unell, I. and Aldgate, J. (1999) *Children's Needs – Parenting Capacity: The Impact of Parental Mental Illness, Problem Alcohol and Drug Use and Domestic Violence on Children's Development*. London: The Stationery Office.

Department of Health (2003) *Every Child Matters*. London: HMSO.

Dobash, R. E. and Dobash, R. P. (1998) *Rethinking Violence Against Women*. London: Sage.

Edleson, J. (1999) Children's witnessing of adult domestic violence. *Journal of Interpersonal Violence* 14(8): 839–870.

Edleson, J. (2002) Studying the co-occurrence of child maltreatment and domestic violence. In S. Graham-Bermann and J. Edleson (eds), *Domestic Violence in the Lives of Children*. Washington, DC: American Psychological Association. pp. 91–110.

Elliot, L., Crombie, I., Irvine, L., Cantrell, J. and Taylor, J. (2001) *Nursing for Health, the Effectiveness of Public Health Nursing: A Review of Systematic Reviews*. Edinburgh: Scottish Executive.

Featherstone, B. and Trinder, L. (1997) Familiar subjects? Domestic violence and child welfare. *Child and Family Social Work* 2: 147–159.

Fitzroy, L. (2001) Violent women: Questions for feminist theory, practice and policy. *Critical Social Policy* 21(1): 7–34.

Gallant, M., Beaulie, M. and Franco, F. (2002) Partnership: An analysis of the concept within the nurse–client relationship. *Journal of Advanced Nursing* 40(2): 149–157.

Gray, B. (2002) Emotional labour and befriending in family support and child protection in Tower Hamlets. *Child and Family Social Work* 7: 13–22.

Greenan, L. (2004) *Violence Against Women: A Literature Review*. Edinburgh: Scottish Executive.

Hanafin, S. (1998) Deconstructing the role of the public health nurse in child protection. *Journal of Advanced Nursing* 28(1): 178–184.

Hartley, C. (2004) Severe domestic violence and child maltreatment: Considering child physical abuse, neglect and failure to protect. *Children and Youth Services Review* 26: 373–392.

Hawkins, D. and Humes, M. (2002) Human rights and domestic violence. *Political Science Quarterly* 117(2): 231–257.

Herrenkohl, T., Sousa, C., Tajima, E., Herrenkohl, R. and Moylan, C. (2008) Intersection of child abuse and exposure to domestic violence. *Trauma Violence Abuse* 9(2): 84–99.

Hester, M., Pearson, C., and Harwin, N. (2000) *Making an Impact: Children and Domestic Violence – A Reader*. London: Jessica Kingsley.

Hochschild, A. R. (1983) *The Managed Heart: Commercialization of Human Feelings*. Berkeley, CA: University of California Press.

Holt, S., Buckley, H. and Whelan, S. (2008) The impact of exposure to domestic violence on children and young people: A review of the literature. *Child Abuse and Neglect* 32: 797–810.

Humphreys, C. (2006) Relevant evidence for practice. In C. Humphreys and N. Stanley (eds), *Domestic Violence and Child Protection Directions for Good Practice*. London and Philadelphia: Jessica Kingsley. pp. 19–32.

Hyland, D. (2002) An exploration of the relationship between patient autonomy and patient advocacy: Implications for nursing. *Nursing Ethics* 9(5): 472–482.

Jouriles, E., McDonald, R., Norwood, W. and Ezell, E. (2000) Issues and controversies in documenting the prevalence of children's exposure to domestic violence. In S. Graham-Bermann and J. Edleson (eds), *Domestic Violence in the Lives of Children: The Future of Research, Intervention and Social Policy*. Washington, DC: American Psychological Association. pp. 13–34.

Kelly, A. and Symonds, A. (2003) *The Social Construction of Community Nursing*. Basingstoke: Palgrave Macmillan.

Lister, P. and Crisp, B. (2005) Clinical supervision in child protection for community nurses. *Child Abuse Review* 14: 57–72.

Mazhindu, D. (2003) Ideal nurses: The social construction of emotional labour. *The European Journal of Psychotherapy, Counselling and Health* 6(3): 243–262.

McGee, C. (2000) Children's and mothers' experiences of support and protection following domestic violence. In J. Hammer, C. Itzin with S. Quaid and D. Wigglesworth (eds), *Home Truths About Domestic Violence: Feminist Influences on Policy and Practice – A Reader*. London: Routledge. pp. 77–95.

Mezey, G. and Bewley, S. (1997) Domestic violence and pregnancy. *BJOG* 104: 528–31.

Mullender, A., Hague, G., Imam, U., Kelly, L., Malos, E. and Regan, L. (2002) *Children's Perspectives on Domestic Violence*. London: Sage.

Osofsky, J. D. (1999) The impact of violence on children. *Domestic Violence and Children* 9(3): Winter: 33–49.

Pask, E. (2001) Nursing responsibility and conditions of practice: Are we justified in holding nurses responsible for their behaviour in situations of patient care? *Nursing Philosophy* 2: 42–52.

Perilla, J., Frndak, K., Lillard, D. and East, C. (2003) A working analysis of the context of learning opportunity and choice. *Violence Against Women* 9(1): 10–46.

Phillips, S. (1996) Labouring the emotions: Expanding the remit of nursing work? *Journal of Advanced Nursing* 24: 139–143.

Powell, C. (2003) Early indicators of child abuse and neglect: A multi-professional Delphi study. *Child Abuse Review* 12: 25–40.

Radford, L. and Hester, M. (2001) Overcoming mother blaming? Future directions for research on mothering and domestic violence. In S. Graham-Bermann and J. Edleson (eds), *Domestic Violence in the Lives of Children*. Washington, DC: American Psychological Association. pp. 135–155.

Radford, L., Corral, S., Bradley, C., Fisher, H., Bassett, C., Howat, N. and Collishaw, S. (2011) *Child Abuse and Neglect in the UK Today*. London: NSPCC. Available at: www.nspcc.org.uk/childstudy (accessed 20 December 2013).

Rodwell, S. (2008) Responding to children who live with domestic abuse: An exploration of the views and experiences of nurses and midwives working in a community setting. Doctoral Thesis, The School of Nursing and Midwifery, University of Dundee.

Royal College of Nursing (2007) *Child Protection, Every Nurse's Responsibility: Guidance for Nursing Staff*. London: RCN.

Russell, D., Springer, K. and Greenfield, E. (2010) Witnessing domestic abuse in childhood as an independent risk factor for depressive symptoms in young adulthood. *Child Abuse and Neglect* 34(6): 448–453.

Sines, D. (2001) The context of community health care nursing. In D. Sines, F. Appleby and E. Raymond (eds), *Community Health Care Nursing*, 2nd edn. Oxford: Blackwell Science. pp. 1–11.

Staden, H. (1998) Alertness to the needs of others: A study of the emotional labour of caring. *Journal of Advanced Nursing* 27: 147–156.

Stanko, E. (1997) Models of understanding violence against women. In S. Bewley, J. Friend and G. Mezey (eds), *Violence Against Women*. London: RCOG Press.

Stanley, N. (1997) Domestic violence and child abuse: Developing practice. *Child and Family Social Work* 2: 135–145.

Stanley, N. (2011) *Children Experiencing Domestic Violence: A Research Review*. Darlington: Research in Practice.

Tarlier, D. S. (2004) Beyond caring: The moral and ethical bases of responsive nurse–patient relationship. *Nursing Philosophy* 5: 230–241.

Tong, R. (1989) *Feminist Thought: A Comprehensive Introduction*. London: Routledge.

Tschudin, V. (2003) *Ethics in Nursing: The Caring Relationship*, 3rd edn. Oxford: Butterworth Heinemann.

Wolak, J. and Finkelhor, D. (1998) Children exposed to partner violence. In J. L. Jasinski and L. M. Williams (eds), *Partner Violence: A Comprehensive Review of 20 Years of Research*. Thousand Oaks, CA: Sage.

Woodtli, M. A. (2000) Domestic violence and the nursing curriculum: Tuning in and tuning up. *Journal of Nursing Education* 39(4): 173–182.

World Health Organization (1978) *International Conference on Primary Care – Alma Ata*. Geneva: WHO.

10

GETTING IT RIGHT: SUPPORTING PROFESSIONAL RESPONSES TO CHILD SAFEGUARDING AND PROTECTION

GILL WATSON AND SANDRA RODWELL

CHAPTER SUMMARY

This text has provided an introductory exploration of a number of theories and practices which impact on the quality of practitioner engagement with the child safeguarding and protection agenda. Theories such as the ecological theory, attachment theory and an assets-based approach have been presented as underpinning the risk assessment process. Set within the context of everyday practice, three key interconnected themes have been discussed: the rights-based agenda, which shapes policy development throughout the United Kingdom and beyond; the roles and responsibilities of practitioners; and the use of an ecological approach to safeguarding children.

A number of recurring aspects of professional practice have been highlighted, underlining the need for specific skills in the assessment process: communication; information gathering; analysis; and taking appropriate action. However, individual practitioners need to understand and be aware of their role and responsibilities and the importance of sharing information regardless of whether or not they work directly with children. A number of factors at an individual practitioner and organisational level have been identified as having the potential to lead to poor practice and the possibility of negative outcomes for children and young people and their families. A lack of awareness, inadequate skill sets and limited support mechanisms within organisations are common themes.

Nonetheless, individual nurses and midwives have to take responsibility for their own professional practice as set out in *The Code: Standards of Conduct, Performance and Ethics for Nurses and Midwives*:

As a professional, you are personally accountable for actions and omissions in your practice and must always be able to justify your decisions. (NMC 2008)

This final chapter begins by providing a summary of the theories, themes and recurring aspects of professional practice. Within this context the concept of emotional labour is introduced before the implications for future developments in relation to nurse education and staff development are discussed. Reference is again made to the application of an ecological framework. This time the framework is used as a means of understanding the influences and relationships between social environmental conditions and the behaviours of individual practitioners and healthcare organisations. This framework does not detract from the professional responsibility of individual practitioners to provide a high standard of practice and care, rather it draws attention to the multiple interrelated factors impacting on practice, and in doing so supports the development of appropriate interventions at each level aimed at mediating the impact of these factors.

This chapter concludes by outlining the importance of organisations and individual practitioners' engagement in the support and supervision process and the implications for nurse education and professional development in relation to the safeguarding agenda.

AIMS OF THIS CHAPTER

This chapter has three aims. The first aim is to summarise the key points identified in the preceding chapters within the context of the three main themes. The second aim is to address elements of professional practice which facilitate or hinder good safeguarding practices from the individual and organisational perspective. The third aim is to introduce the conceptual ecological framework and its application as a tool for identifying and addressing at an individual and organisational level the support needs of nurses and midwives in their professional response to the child safeguarding agenda.

Learning outcomes

After reading this chapter and following a period of reflection, the reader will be able to:

- Identify and discuss the necessary qualities, such as knowledge, skills and emotional abilities, required by practitioners to work with children, young people and their families.
- Identify and discuss the multiple levels of influence on practice development.
- Understand the importance of applying an ecological framework to the analysis of the response of nurses and midwives to child protection in practice at an organisational and individual practitioner level.
- Reflect critically on their safeguarding practices and those of the wider practice community.

Key words

ecological model; emotional intelligence; practice development; professional practice; support and supervision;

A SUMMARY OF THE KEY THEMES

Rights-based agenda and child-centred care

The political responses to child welfare have changed over the last 50 years in parallel with the positioning of children in our society, mainly facilitated through the rights-based agenda. Child welfare is now considered in much wider terms than before, incorporating the broad concept of safeguarding as well as child protection. The resulting changes in legislation and policies across the United Kingdom makes explicit the responsibilities of parents and other carers, including nurses and midwives, towards children, making their developmental needs and welfare paramount in meeting what must be considered 'the best interests of the child'. It is now accepted that children and young people should expect to have their views, experiences and preferences, as expressed by themselves, listened to and acted upon.

It is now understood that all practitioners have a professional responsibility to safeguard children, and this is clearly set out in the Nursing and Midwifery Council Guidelines (NMC 2008). In line with this responsibility, individual practitioners should be familiar with the policies and processes regarding the safeguarding of children and young people within their local area.

Practice delivery is shaped through the application of a public health approach (Barlow and Calam 2011) which adopts an ecological framework to assess and analyse the potential risk or vulnerability of children and young people, before early evidence-based interventions are introduced, to address child-centred needs. The use of the ecologically based assessment framework My World Assessment Triangle, as discussed in Chapter 6 is one example of this approach which is applied in practice by professionals from various disciplines and organisations. Applying an assets-based analysis to this process helps the individual practitioner or multi-disciplinary team focus on the protective factors rather than the negative aspects of the child or young person's environment, as discussed in Chapter 5. An important asset when assessing risk is that of attachment, as set out in Chapter 3. It is argued that the nature of the relationship of the child or young person with their main caregiver or other significant people around them is an important part of the risk assessment process.

Within the context of the three themes are a number of recurring aspects of professional practice identified throughout this introductory text which are central to an effective and efficient response of individual practitioners to meet the safeguarding agenda.

RECURRING ASPECTS OF PROFESSIONAL PRACTICE

The importance of effective communication, comprehensive information gathering, analysis and appropriate action have been discussed and illustrated throughout this text, using practice-based examples. At the same time the need for practitioners to critically reflect on these processes and their application of them has been set out.

The discourse associated with nursing practice with an emphasis on partnership working, the nurse–client relationship, a holistic approach to care and autonomy for the client has been discussed. The possibility that these aspects of professional practice can both direct and constrain practice has been introduced in Chapter 7 within the context of family-centred care, and in Chapter 9 with its focus on domestic abuse in the lives of children.

The process of establishing and maintaining a partnership based on trust and mutual respect requires the practitioner to draw on the psychological, social and practical dimensions of nursing care. Within the context of safeguarding children, these aspects of the process may lead the practitioner to experience a degree of conflict and tension as they consider the needs of the family, their client who may be an adult or a child, and any children or young people within in the family. Central to these dimensions of care is the need for practitioners to manage the range of emotions they may experience, reflecting the concept of emotional labour as outlined in Chapter 9.

While there is evidence of good professional nursing and midwifery practice in safeguarding and protecting children and young people as well as measured approaches in the use of early interventions to support families, unsatisfactory reports claiming practices of poor quality have also been identified. The Laming Report of the Victoria Climbié Inquiry (Laming 2003) and reviews into child protection (Lord Laming 2009; Munro 2011) further confirm the limitations in the practices of healthcare practitioners. Evidenced within this introductory text is the need for education because of low levels of knowledge and skills, poor inter-professional working patterns (Sidebotham and the ALSPAC Study Team 2006; Brandon et al. 2010), compounded by competing agendas (Crisp and Lister 2004), limited experience in the area of child protection and lack of emotional support (Piltz and Wachtel 2010). Recognition of the emotional aspect of care has implications for nurse education and practice development.

EMOTIONAL LABOUR

Building on a previous study of emotional labour and nursing undertaken by Smith (1992), Smith and Gray (2001) explored the content and process of emotional labour within the context of nursing students and the nurse education environment. Smith and Gray concluded that emotional labour is a routine part of nursing. However, as highlighted in Chapter 9, there have been a number of studies which suggest that this aspect of practice is neglected. This situation may have potentially negative consequences for practitioners and their clients. This conclusion appears to be borne out by the work of Warne and McAndrew (2005).

As part of a larger study, Warne and McAndrew (2005) explored the extent to which mental health nurses were prepared and able to work with adult clients who had experienced of childhood sexual abuse. Through a review of the published literature they explored the impact on the nurse–client relationship of nurses themselves having experience of childhood sexual abuse. The authors identified a number of underlying factors which shaped the response of mental health nurses at a personal level, for example personal values, beliefs and personal experiences. This was inclusive of the opportunity to address their own experiences of childhood sexual abuse or to explore their personal attitudes and beliefs.

Providing practitioners with appropriate support on a number of levels was considered as a means of improving the care nurses would then give to their clients (Warne and McAndrew 2005). The authors referred to a mixture of initiatives aimed at supporting staff in undertaking their professional responsibilities as a 'holding environment' (2005: 684). The authors conclude by stating:

> for those involved in delivering mental health services and who are not able to access this type of holding environment it could be argued we are setting people up to fail. (2005: 684)

It is not unreasonable to apply this sentiment to all practitioners and their response to the safeguarding children and young people agenda. It is a false dichotomy to suggest that practitioners do not have similar concerns and experiences to their clients and it is important to recognise that these may impact either consciously or unconsciously on their practice. It is possible that the emotional charge which is always there or there-abouts in safeguarding and protection work has a negative impact on practice because the emotional feelings of nurses and midwives receive very little attention or consideration.

IMPLICATIONS FOR NURSE EDUCATION AND DEVELOPMENT

Although not couched in such terms, the need for a 'holding environment' was explored in the work of Smith and Gray (2001). The important role of link lecturers and mentors in providing an appropriate environment for nursing students to explore their emotional response to situations they come across in practice was highlighted. Student nurses talked positively about being able to share and discuss their experiences with others in a meaningful way. The authors conclude that the concept of emotional labour needs to be grounded in nurse education and practice in a formal systematic way. The need for emotional labour to be acknowledged and not 'ignored or exploited' is expressed (Smith and Gray 2001: 236). The authors also identify the need to develop an appropriate format for recording how emotional labour manifests itself at an individual and practice level in order for it to be incorporated into education and practice.

It is concerning to note that the more recent findings of Piltz and Wachtel (2010) regarding the lack of emotional support have not experienced a great deal of discussion or interest in research terms.

Reflective activity

Take some time to consider a situation you have encountered where you have had to manage an emotional response in order to provide the necessary 'professional' nursing response. Consider the following:

- Did you speak to anyone about this experience?
- If yes, what was it you hoped to gain from sharing your experience?
- Did it help?
- What lessons did you take from this experience?
- If you did not speak to anyone about your experience, how did you feel afterwards?
- What would have been helpful?

PREPARING FOR CHANGE

The accumulation of evidence highlights the need for change to the present systems and processes used to prepare practitioners. Competency frameworks have been helpful in setting out the level of knowledge, skills, and, some would argue, capabilities, required for differing levels of practitioner within the healthcare workforce. Competency assessments have been used within nursing and midwifery clinical education for some time to evaluate learners. However, there remain on-going debates as to their place in the education of practitioners (Gardner et al. 2008). A common feature of competency frameworks is the apparent fixation with knowledge and skills, but often missing or shrouded in an ambiguous way is the impact of emotional competence, conceptualised through levels of empathy, understanding and the ability to identify another person's perspective. Such qualities have often been considered synonymous with the job of nursing (Smith and Gray 2001).

Together, the evidence from research, reports and reviews and the main themes evolving from the earlier chapters presented in this book would suggest that competency frameworks, on their own, are insufficient in guiding the preparation of nursing and midwifery practitioners to address safeguarding and child protection effectively in practice. Applying the all-encompassing concept of practice development is perhaps what is required. Arguably, the cognitive abilities, behaviours and experiences of the practitioner are more effective when embedded within a culture with a shared meaning of values, beliefs, attitudes and expectation starting from recruitment to undergraduate education through to post-qualifying practice (Manley 2004).

A FRAMEWORK FOR SUPPORTING NURSES AND MIDWIVES TO SAFEGUARD CHILDREN, YOUNG PEOPLE AND THEIR FAMILIES

The purpose of this section is to introduce a theoretical approach to guide professional practice development of nurses and midwives to facilitate the safeguarding and protection of children, young people and their families. Arguably, to achieve this outcome, practice development requires being proactive, systematic and evidence-based.

Practice development

The overall purpose of practice development is to develop patient-centred care into an effective concern operationalised through changing the culture and context in which care is provided (McCormack and Garbett 2004). Garbett and McCormack (2002) offer this definition:

> Practice development is a continuous process of improvement towards increased effectiveness in patient-centred care. This is brought about by helping healthcare teams to develop their knowledge and skills and to transform the culture and context of care. It is enabled and supported by facilitators committed to systematic, rigorous continuous processes of emancipatory change that reflect the perspective of service users. (2002: 88)

Applying this definition to nursing and midwifery practitioners working towards safeguarding children and young people in the context of their families highlights the need for a multi-level approach. This does not take away the responsibilities of individual organisations or practitioners but recognises the impact of multi-agency interaction and social welfare policy-makers in meeting professional standards in the care of children, young people and their families. What it does offer is a clear direction for development of all services that contribute to safeguarding and protective care. However, providing a structure and identifying the multiple processes to change practice requires a conceptual strategy or framework to ensure that all levels and conditions can be identified and addressed. Adopting an ecological perspective would facilitate a multi-level view of the contextual influences shaping the professional response of nurses and midwives to the safeguarding and protection agenda.

The ecological framework is one such theoretical approach which has often been used to address dynamic interactions and influences involving relationships, the environments in which they develop and human behaviours. As discussed in Chapter 4, Bronfenbrenner (1979) was one of the first to conceptualise an ecological framework originally to explore, evaluate and explain the dynamic influences to human development. Bronfenbrenner's conceptual framework viewed behaviour as being shaped by multiple levels of influence, with each level representing a social influence or environment. Bronfenbrenner labelled each social influence or environment according to their position and level of representation, such as micro-, meso-, exo- and macrosystem.

In more recent times adaptations of Bronfenbrenner's ecological framework have been use to explain a number of issues or activities, such as health promotion (McLeroy et al. 1988), nurses' attitudes to survivors of domestic violence (Woodtli 2000), intimate partner violence (Little and Kantor 2002), child maltreatment (Sidebotham et al. 2006) and health behaviours (Sallis et al. 2008). With each adaptation, the characteristics of the individual within the microsystem change and the characteristics of the other system also change accordingly. What does not change, however, is that each layer of influence continues to impact on behaviour of the individual, which in turn impacts on the other systems. A major strength, therefore, of Bronfenbrenner's conceptualised ecological framework is the remarkable flexibility it offers to address differing problems, conditions or issues, as highlighted above.

Ecological framework supporting practice development

Garbett and McCormack's (2002) definition of practice development identifies the contextual processes required to change practice. While these processes are essential to support change, it is the ultimate outcome of behaviour from individuals, organisations, multi-agency working and social welfare policy makers which is used to judge or measure overall effectiveness. Applying this to nursing and midwifery practitioners, it is the behaviours of individual practitioners, their working within a multi-agency environment, the wider organisational culture and social welfare policies directing practice that are deemed either satisfactory or unsatisfactory by the quality of behaviour responses to the child protection agenda. The quality of the multi-level interaction and environment therefore impacts on behaviour outcomes.

Table 10.1 Four levels of influence on behaviour of the individual practitioner
and the organisation

Level	Type of influence
Microsystem	*Intrapersonal factors*: individual factors such as developmental history education; self-efficacy; attitudes; behaviours; experience.
Mesosystem	*Interpersonal factors*: formal and informal social networks within and outwith work; social support from family.
Exosystem	*Organisational factors*: culture; formal and informal networks; rules and expectations; structures and processes, including supervision; relationships with other professional groups, such as Higher Institutions of Educations (HIE); other universal services.
Macrosystem	*Policies and legislation*: legislation, policies and professional bodies such as the NMC.

The interaction and environmental conditions in which individuals, multi-agency partnerships and organisations engage suggest that the conceptual ecological framework is well suited in guiding practice development change as well as analysing outcomes of change.

Applying the principles underpinning an ecological framework to practice development and the safeguarding agenda, four layers of influence are identified (see Table 10.1).

ALIGNING LEVELS OF INFLUENCE TO PRACTICE DEVELOPMENT

In Table 10.1, four theoretical levels of influence on practice development are presented. The application of each level to highlight the impact on practice development to support the child safeguarding and protection agenda is now considered.

Figure 10.1 presents the four interrelated levels of influence on nursing and midwifery professional practice.

Individual practitioner (microsystems)

In the centre of the conceptual ecological model is the practitioner. The characteristics of the practitioner are significant in shaping their ability to develop in their practice environment. The practitioner's individual developmental history has evolved through their past experiences, starting very early in life as discussed in Chapter 3 on attachment. Specific experience of child maltreatment, either personally or someone in close proximity, may influence the practitioner's professional response in practice, as discussed earlier in this chapter.

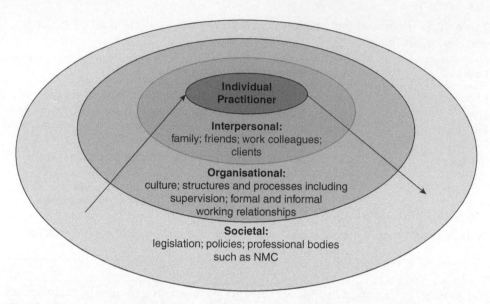

Figure 10.1   Four interrelated levels of influence on nursing and midwifery practice

The practitioner needs specific skills in order to address the needs of children, young people and their families. These require development across undergraduate and post-qualifying education, including: identified skills of communication; building relationships and working partnerships; critical reflection and analytical skills; and knowledge relating to child development. Knowledge and understanding of professional regulation shaped by legislation, policies and professional codes (macrosystem) of practice are also required. The practitioner is accountable and responsible for their practice. They need to communicate their needs to their employing organisation (exosystem). Equally, the organisation is required to support development, including emotional support, to enable the practitioner to fulfil their responsibilities.

Reflective activity

Reflecting on your own professional attributes, identify those that make you the practitioner you are today.

Informal/formal social and professional networks (mesosystem)

The second layer of influence comprises social networks, formal and informal, which are recognised as contributing to the individual practitioner's values and belief systems. This again is related to developmental experiences witnessed within relationships with others including their family and friends, as well as work colleagues, other professional colleagues and clients and their families. This level of interaction and social environment is a powerful medium for influencing behaviour, including the need for change or not as the case may be (mesosystem).

A combination of factors from the intrapersonal and interpersonal can indeed influence the degree of practitioner and practice cohesion as well as to whether inter-professional and inter-agency working is successful at the point of front-line practice.

Institutions/organisations (exosystem)

The third layer of influence is the employing healthcare organisation. This was highlighted earlier in this chapter as having a responsibility to support practitioners in their preparation for their safeguarding roles and responsibilities. Specifically, emotional support needs to have a high priority. Equally, practitioners also have a responsibility to identify and communicate their needs for future development in order that they can fulfil their roles in practice.

This level of influence incorporates multi-agency working at a strategic level. Individual professional practice is influenced by the culture of the employing organisation and the organisation's relationship with partner organisations.

Healthcare organisations make a major contribution to the undergraduate recruitment programmes in partnership with higher education institutions (HEIs). Identifying potential recruits with the fundamental attributes and abilities impacts on the quality of future nursing and midwifery practices. Both healthcare organisations and HEIs contribute to the assessment of knowledge, emotional competence and skills of student practitioners throughout educational programmes. A major influence on learning in practice is the quality of mentorship in the clinical environment.

Rycroft-Malone (2004) states that in order to change into a learning environment, an organisation must consider four specific areas, briefly described below:

- *Context*: requires appropriate and transparent systems and processes regarding decision making, information, feedback, power and authority.
- *Culture*: defined by organisational beliefs and values; promotion of a learning environment; values individuals and client base; rewards, values and recognises good practice; values relationships with others and team working.
- *Leadership*: requires the ability to transform the context and culture of the organisation from 'command and control' to one which is evidence-based and where everyone is recognised as a leader in some capacity. This type of leader proposes and works towards a shared vision. Transformational leaders are emotionally competent, empathic, motivational, inspirational, reflective, facilitative and empowering, and self-confident.
- *Evaluation*: measuring practice requires a framework to ensure that evidence is gathered from multiple levels or sources using both qualitative and quantitative methods. Such a framework explores context, culture and leadership through the exploration of user experiences and practice narratives and reflections (McCormack et al. 2002) as well as the statistics relating to outcomes.

Reflective activity

Take some time to reflect on the organisational environment in which you practice. Can you identify the characteristics of the context, culture, leadership and evaluation which impact on the effectiveness of safeguarding children, young people and their families in practice?

Government and professional policies (macrosystem)

The fourth level of influence comprises social welfare policies, either from government, conventions or professional bodies such as the NMC. Influencing this level are the international and national agendas regarding social welfare, for example the rights-based agenda. Wider societal beliefs and values as expressed through voting in local or general elections, as well as through other means common to a democratic country, are influential at this level.

In Chapter 1, we presented a review of policies informed through legislation which were responsible for changing the roles and responsibilities of practitioners in meeting the child safeguarding and protection agenda. The European Convention on Human Rights (1950) and the United Nations Convention on the Rights of the Child (1989) significantly influenced the change in policy direction. Such policies significantly impact and inform the activities of healthcare organisations and how they relate in practice with other professional organisations which ultimately lead to changes in the practice provided by front-line services.

A further influence on organisation and the practice of individual nurses or midwives is the Nursing and Midwifery Council (NMC). The NMC's policies on practice are set out in what is termed 'The Code'. The Code makes explicit the professional standards of conduct, performance and ethics for nurses and midwives (NMC 2008), and provides clear direction as to acceptable and ethical professional standards for practice to safeguard and protect all members of the public.

This conceptualised ecological framework clearly highlights the levels and direction of influence contributing to practice development supporting and facilitating child safeguarding and protection practices. It is therefore important that health and social care organisations, educators, students and trained practitioners apply this framework when critically appraising the different aspects of their service or practice in order to identify strengths and deficit in their practice. Legislation and policies clearly set the direction of care. Putting policy into practice requires adequate resources. The main resource for an organisation is its practitioners. Engaging in meaningful support and supervision as a 'holding environment' is a critical aspect of training and development so that practitioners can engage appropriately in the safeguarding agenda and children and young people and their families receive the support they require.

CLINICAL SUPERVISION

Government guidance suggests that all healthcare practitioners should have access to regular clinical supervision sessions. Effective supervision is considered necessary to facilitate continuous professional development. Clinical supervision is defined by the Royal College of Nursing as

> an activity that brings skilled supervisors and practitioners together in order to reflect upon their practice. It is a time for nurses and midwives to think about their knowledge and skills and to consider development to improve care. (2013)

The principles of supervision are to facilitate practice development through a process of reflection and discussion to improve standards of care.

An integrated review of the literature exploring the barriers to nurses reporting suspected cases of child abuse and neglect found that the lack of emotional support for nurses was one of the influencing factors which reduced the likelihood of positive outcomes for children and their families (Piltz and Wachtel 2010). The lack of support appears to compound other factors identified at different levels which shape their behaviour, in particular working with other agencies in a formal manner in relation to addressing suspicions of child abuse and neglect. Effective and regular clinical supervision has the potential to mediate the negative behaviours of practitioners. Organisations have a responsibility to children, young people and their families to ensure that the services they access are appropriate, timely and effective. Good governance would suggest that a supported, educated and professional approach to the safeguarding agenda requires an educated and supported workforce. Effective regular supervision should be a priority if the organisations delivering healthcare are to meet their obligations.

CONCLUSION

In this final chapter we have brought together and summarised the interconnected themes that have been discussed throughout this introductory book. A number of professional aspects of practice have been identified as central to managing the response of nurses and midwives to the safeguarding and protecting children and young people agenda. At the same time, an important part of professional practice which rarely receives much attention has also been identified: the emotional aspects of front-line practice when working with children, young people and families.

While competency frameworks have been a constant element of nurse and midwifery education for some time, they are insufficient on their own to guide professional practice development. An ecological framework has been presented as a means of understanding the differing levels of influence on practice development. Highlighted throughout this chapter are the responsibilities of individual practitioners and those of the wider organisation to prepare nurses and midwives for their roles and responsibilities in safeguarding and protecting children, young people and their families.

FURTHER READING

Gray, B. (2002) Emotional labour and befriending in family support and child protection in Tower Hamlets. *Child and Family Social Work* 7: 13–22.

REFERENCES

Barlow, J. and Calam, R. (2011) A public health approach to safeguarding in the 21st century. *Child Abuse Review* 20: 238–255.

Brandon, M., Sidebotham, P., Balley, S. and Belderson, P. (2010) *A Study of Recommendations Arising from Serious Case Reviews 2009–2010*. London: Department for Education.

Bronfenbrenner, U. (1979) *The Ecology of Human Development: Experiments by Nature and Design*. London: Harvard University Press.

Crisp, B. and Lister, P. (2004) Child protection and public health nurse's responsibilities. *Journal of Advanced Nursing* 476: 656–665.

European Convention on Human Rights (1950) *Convention for the Protection of Human Rights and Fundamental Freedoms in Rights*. Strasbourg: European Court of Human Rights.

Garbett, R. and McCormack, B. (2002) A concept analysis of practice development. *Nursing Times Research* 7(2): 87–100.

Gardner, A., Hase, S., Gardner, G., Dunn, S. and Carryer, J. (2008) From competence to capability: A study of nurse practitioners in clinical practice. *Journal of Clinical Nursing* 17: 250–258.

Laming, Lord (2003) *The Victoria Climbié Inquiry*. London: The Stationery Office.

Laming, Lord (2009) *The Protection of Children in England: A Progress Report*. London: The Stationery Office.

Little, L. and Kantor, G. (2002) Using ecological theory to understand intimate partner violence and child maltreatment. *Journal of Community Health Nursing* 19(3): 133–145.

Manley, K. (2004) Transformational culture: A culture of effectiveness. In B. McCormack, K. Manley and R. Garbett (eds), *Practice Development in Nursing*. Oxford: Blackwell.

McCormack, B. and Garbett, R. (2004) A concept analysis of practice development. In B. McCormack, K. Manley, and K. Garbett, R. (eds), *Practice Development in Nursing*. Oxford: Blackwell.

McCormack, B., Manley, K. and Garbett, R. (eds) (2002) *Practice Development in Nursing*. Oxford: Blackwell.

McLeroy, K., Bibeau, D., Steckler, A. and Glanz, K. (1988) An ecological perspective on health promotion programmes. *Health Education Quarterly* 15(4): 351–377.

Munro, E. (2011) *The Munro Review of Child Protection: Final Report*. London: Department for Education.

Nursing and Midwifery Council (NMC) (2008) *The Code: Standards of Conduct, Performance and Ethics for Nurses and Midwives*. London: NMC. Available at: www.nmc-uk.org/Publications/Standards/ (accessed January 2013).

Piltz, A. and Wachtel, T. (2010) Barriers that inhibit nurses reporting suspected cases of child abuse and neglect. *Australian Journal of Advanced Nursing* 26(3): 93–100.

Royal College of Nursing (2013) *Clinical Supervision*. London: RCN. Available at: www.rcn.org.uk/support/rcn_direct_online_advice/a-z2/clinical_supervision/clinical_supervision (accessed August 2013).

Rycroft-Malone, J. (2004) Research implementation evidence, context and facilitation – the PARIHS framework. In B. McCormack, K. Manley and R. Garbett (eds), *Practice Development in Nursing*. Oxford: Blackwell. pp. 118–147.

Sallis, J., Owen, N. and Fisher, E. (2008) Ecological models of health behaviour. In K. Glanz, B.K. Rimer and K. Viswanath (eds), *Health Behaviour and Health Education Theory, Research and Practice*. San Francisco, CA: Jossey-Bass.

Sidebotham, P. and the ALSPAC Study Team (2006) Patterns of child abuse in early childhood, a cohort study of the 'children of the nineties'. *Child Abuse Review* 9: 311–320.

Smith, P. (1992) *The Emotional Labour of Nursing*. London: Macmillan.

Smith, P. and Gray, B. (2001) Reassessing the concept of emotional labour in student nurse education: Role of link lecturers and mentors in a time of change. *Nursing Education Today* 21: 230–237.

United Nations (1989) *United Nations Convention on the Rights of the Child*. Geneva: United Nations.

Warne, T. and McAndrew, S. (2005) The shackles of abuse: Unprepared to work at the edge of reason. *Journal of Psychiatric and Mental Health Nursing* 12: 679–686.

Woodtli, A. (2000) Domestic violence and the nursing curriculum: Tuning in and tuning up. *Journal of Nursing Education* 39(4): 173–182.

INDEX